Dealing With The Menopause

Your Roadmap to Understand the Three Stages of Hormonal Shifts, Build a Strong Support Network, and Manage Symptoms Through Simple Lifestyle Solutions

Annabel Wave

Table of Contents

Introduction

If you've ever found yourself silently whispering to your body, "What in the world is happening to me?" you're not alone. Menopause, dear reader, is like a second puberty no one prepared us for. It knocks on our doors with a suitcase full of surprises—hot flashes, mood swings, and midnight musings about whether it's possible to install a personal mini air conditioner under our shirts. But here's the heartening news: menopause isn't a medical condition to tiptoe around in hushed tones. It's a natural, albeit cheeky, phase of life that, believe it or not, we can navigate with grace, confidence, and a few laughs along the way.

That's where I step in—your empathetic guide through the meandering pathways of menopause. My passion? To arm you and those who walk this journey with you with reputable, easy-to-understand guidance that lightens the load. Whether you're in the thick of it, see it on the horizon, or are supporting someone who's navigating these waters, I'm here to educate and empower. Together, we'll build a supportive community where no one feels they must whisper about their hot flashes.

This book is more than just words on a page. It promises to demystify menopause, blending scientific explanations with personal testimonies and sprinkling in holistic lifestyle solutions like a well-seasoned dish. The goal? To empower you to feel informed, supported, and part of a larger community that gets it. No one should have to go through this feeling of isolation or lack of information.

And here's the thing - while the primary audience might be those of us experiencing menopause firsthand, this book throws its doors wide open. Partners, family members, friends—you're all invited. This is a comprehensive resource for anyone touched by the menopause journey, eager to under- stand, support, and walk alongside their loved ones.

This book fully understands menopause and offers actionable advice on lifestyle solutions, emotional support, and community building. Expect a mix of scientific backing and personal stories that illuminate the realities of menopause. From diet and exercise to stress management and finding your tribe, we're covering it all, comprehensively addressing the physical, emotional, and psychological aspects.

Let me share a snippet from my journey—there was a time when I thought a hot flash was something only experienced in the tropics. Fast-forward to my first, shall we say, personal summer moment in the middle of a snowstorm, and boy, was I wrong. We'll tackle these common misconceptions and challenges together, laughing and learning our way through.

This book champions a holistic approach to managing menopause by incorporating various strategies, holistic twist, and blending bioidentical hormones, HRT, testosterone, and natural herbs. It's not just about salads and squats; it's about embracing your body, mind, and spirit in a supportive community. Like a custom-tailored suit, these approaches aim to fit you just right, waving goodbye to those pesky hormone imbalances with a sprinkle of humor and a dash of science.

So, I invite you, dear reader, to dive into this book with an open heart and a curious mind. Let's explore every avenue, traditional and alternative, to manage menopause. Become an advocate for your health and well-being, equipped with knowledge, strategies, and a good dose of humor.

By the end of this journey, I promise you a transformation. Menopause will no longer loom as a phase of uncertainty and discomfort but will emerge as a time of empowerment and well-being. Let's change the narrative and make this chapter one of the most fulfilling yet. Welcome to the ride of your life—buckle up; it will be enlightening and, dare I say, a bit fun!

1

Exploring the Scientific Aspects of Menopause

When the noise of everyday living settles into a soft hum in the quiet moments of a woman's life, she might notice the subtle yet profound shifts occurring within her body. These shifts are not sudden or explosive; instead, they unfold with the slow grace of a day melting into night. This is menopause, a natural biological process that marks a significant phase in a woman's life. Unlike the onset of puberty, which often arrives with unmistakable changes, menopause can begin its approach so gently that it's almost a whisper.

1.1 The Science of Menopause

Understanding the biological underpinnings of menopause is akin to learning a new language—one that explains the whispers and the roars of our bodies as they navigate this inevitable transition. Menopause is not merely a halt in menstrual cycles; it is a complex, multifaceted shift that encompasses the entire body, influenced by the intricate dance of hormones within.

At its core, menopause signifies the cessation of ovulation, a milestone medically recognized after twelve consecutive months without a menstrual period. This pause in menstruation is not a disorder but a natural stage in a woman's life, signifying the end of her reproductive years. The mechanics of this transition are orchestrated by the ovaries, which gradually reduce the production of estrogen and progesterone. These hormones have played leading roles throughout a woman's reproductive life, not only facilitating menstruation and pregnancy but also influencing a myriad of bodily functions.

The transition through menopause is typically divided into three stages: perimenopause, menopause, and post- menopause. Perimenopause, often unnoticed at first, heralds the beginning of this transition. During this stage, women may start to experience irregular menstrual cycles, a direct result of fluctuating hormone levels. It's a time of change that can span several years, during which the symptoms commonly associated with menopause begin to surface.

The following perimenopause is menopause itself, defined by the complete cessation of menstrual periods for one full year. During this stage, the ovaries significantly reduce hormone production, leading to the absence of ovulation and menstruation. Finally, post-menopause marks the period after menopause, encompassing the rest of a woman's life. Hormone levels stabilize at a lower level, but the impact of these changes continues to resonate throughout the body.

The effects of declining hormone levels extend far beyond the reproductive system. Estrogen, for example, plays a crucial role in maintaining bone density, regulating cholesterol, and supporting skin health. Its reduction can lead to an increased risk of osteoporosis, cardiovascular disease, and changes in skin elasticity. Similarly, progesterone's decline can affect sleep patterns, mood, and the body's response to insulin. Understanding these effects is pivotal, as it underscores the systemic nature of menopause—a transition that influences physical, emotional, and cognitive well-being.

Consider the impact of these hormonal changes on daily life in a real-life scenario. A woman in her late 40s notices her once clockwork-like menstrual cycle becoming unpredictable. She may experience hot flashes at inopportune moments, such as during an important presentation or during a family dinner. Once taken for granted, sleep becomes elusive, with night sweats disrupting her rest and affecting her mood and concentration the next day. This scenario is not uncommon, and it highlights the broad- reaching implications of the hormonal shifts occurring during menopause.

Equipping oneself with knowledge is essential for navigating transitions effectively. Understanding the science of menopause provides a foundation upon which to build strategies for managing symptoms and maintaining quality of life. It empowers women to make informed decisions about their health, seeking interventions that align with their needs and preferences. Whether through lifestyle adjustments, hormone therapy, or alternative treatments, the goal is to support the body and mind through this natural yet challenging phase.

As we delve deeper into the nuances of menopause, remember that knowledge is power. By comprehensively understanding the biological process, the role of hormones, and the stages of menopause, women can confidently approach this phase, prepared to tackle its challenges head- on. This chapter serves as the first step in demystifying menopause, laying the groundwork for a journey marked not by fear or uncertainty but by informed action and self- compassion.

1.2 Symptoms and Their Variability

In the tapestry of menopause, each woman stitches her unique pattern, weaving threads of symptoms that vary in color, intensity, and texture. This variability underscores the profoundly personal nature of menopause, where one's experience can diverge significantly from another's. It is this spectrum of symptoms, ranging from the mildly inconvenient to the profoundly disruptive, that paints the complex picture of the menopausal transition.

Hot flashes are one of the most emblematic symptoms, a sudden warmth permeating the body, often accompanied by a flushed face and sweating. Imagine standing in a serene, cool stream only to be unexpectedly enveloped by a wave of heat;

this juxtaposition captures the essence of a hot flash. For some, this sensation is a rare inconvenience, a brief reminder of the body's shifting hormonal landscape. For others, it's a frequent and intense disruption, a wave that crashes over them multiple times daily, challenging their comfort and composure.

Night sweats, the nocturnal counterpart to hot flashes, disrupt the sanctuary of sleep, drenching nightclothes and bedding in sweat. This intrusion into rest can fray the edges of one's patience and resilience, turning restorative sleep into a nightly battle against the body's unpredictable thermostat. Mood changes weave through the menopausal experience as well, with some women finding themselves on a rollercoaster of emotions, their moods shifting as swiftly and unpredictably as the wind. The once familiar landscape of their emotional well-being now feels like uncharted territory, marked by sudden tears or irritation at the slightest provocation.

Vaginal dryness, less frequently discussed but equally impactful, adds another layer to the complexity of menopause. It speaks to the intimate nature of the changes affecting relationships, self-esteem, and sexual health. Often shrouded in silence, this symptom can carry a weight of isolation, a quiet reminder of the body's internal shifts.

The severity of these symptoms varies widely, influenced by a confluence of factors, including lifestyle, health, and even attitude. For some, a healthy diet, regular exercise, and stress management techniques provide a buffer against the more disruptive symptoms, mitigating their impact and enhancing quality of life. These proactive measures can act like a balm, soothing the rough edges of menopause and restoring a measure of control over one's body and well-being.

Conversely, individuals with chronic health conditions or limited access to healthcare may find menopause exacerbates their existing challenges. Symptoms can become more intense, transforming menopause into a magnified obstacle course. However, attitude plays a crucial role; viewing menopause as a manageable phase of life can significantly ease navigation through its symptoms, with a positive mindset guiding resilience and grace.

This variability demands a personalized approach to management that acknowledges the unique interplay of factors affecting each woman. It challenges the notion of a one-size-fits-all solution, advocating for strategies tailored to individual needs, preferences, and circumstances. It calls for open, honest conversations with healthcare providers, a willingness to explore a range of management options, and, perhaps most importantly, a compassionate understanding of one's own body and its transitions.

Recognizing the diversity of menopausal experiences also offers an opportunity for connection and support. Sharing stories and strategies can illuminate the common threads that bind these experiences while honoring individual differences. It can foster a sense of community, a collective acknowledgment that while the journey through menopause is personal, no one needs to navigate it in isolation.

The landscape of menopause, with its wide range of symptoms and experiences, reflects the broader diversity of women's lives and health. It underscores the importance of a nuanced understanding of menopause, which respects the complexity of women's bodies and their capacity for adaptation and resilience. In this light, menopause can be seen not as a uniform challenge to overcome but as a multifaceted transition to be navigated, offering opportunities for growth, understanding, and connection.

1.3 Hormonal Fluctuations and Their Impact

In the realm of menopause, estrogen and progesterone act as the conductors of an orchestra, guiding the symphony of the body through rhythms both harmonious and discordant. As these hormone levels ebb and flow, their influence extends far beyond the reproductive system, orchestrating a series of changes that ripple through the body and mind. This section illuminates the profound impact of these fluctuations, revealing the depth of their reach and the breadth of their effects.

Estrogen, once the linchpin of reproductive health, sees its levels fluctuate wildly during Perimenopause before their eventual decline. This reduction is not a quiet fade but a disruption that reverberates, affecting various systems within the body. Bone density, for example, feels the absence of estrogen acutely. This hormone plays a critical role in the maintenance and renewal of bone tissue; without its protective effects, the process of bone resorption accelerates, leading to a decrease in bone mass and an increased risk of fractures.

Women, now standing on the precipice of post-menopause, find themselves confronting the reality of osteoporosis, a condition characterized by porous, weakened bones.

The heart, too, long shielded by the effects of estrogen, finds itself more vulnerable in the face of declining hormone levels. Estrogen's departure leaves a void in its wake, with cardiovascular health now compromised. This hormone once facilitated a favorable lipid profile, encouraging the presence of high-density lipoprotein (HDL) cholesterol while keeping low-density lipoprotein (LDL) cholesterol at bay. Its influence extended to the vasculature, fostering flexibility in the arteries and promoting healthy blood flow. The decline in estrogen shifts this balance, paving the way for increased cholesterol levels, hypertension, and a stiffer cardiovascular system—factors that collectively heighten the risk of heart disease.

The canvas of menopause is painted not only with these physical changes but with strokes that color the realm of emotional and cognitive health. Estrogen and progesterone, in their prime, contributed to neurotransmitter regulation, affecting mood, emotion, and cognition. With their decline, the curtain rises on a stage set for mood swings, irritability, and episodes of melancholy. Memory, too, may falter, with women reporting instances of forgetfulness or a nebulous feeling of cognitive fog. This intertwining of hormonal balance and mental health underscores the complexity of menopause, where the physical cannot be extricated from the psychological.

As the narrative unfolds, long-term health considerations demand attention. The specter of osteoporosis looms large, with its potential to compromise independence and quality of life. Here, the dialogue expands to include strategies for bone health preservation, from calcium and vitamin D supplementation to weight-bearing exercises designed to fortify the skeletal framework. Similarly, post-menopause's increased risk of cardiovascular disease necessitates a proactive approach to heart health, advocating regular physical activity, a heart-healthy diet, and monitoring of blood pressure and cholesterol levels.

This landscape, marked by hormonal fluctuations and their far-reaching impact, invites a nuanced understanding of menopause. It is a period characterized not by loss but by transformation, where adaptation becomes the key to navigating the shifts within. In its wisdom, the body continues to communicate; its signals are now a guide to nurturing health and well-being in the face of change.

1.4 The Early Signs: Recognizing Perimenopause

The onset of Perimenopause is akin to the first subtle strokes of dawn, where the night's depth begins to surrender to the light. Yet, both coexist for a time, intermingling in a delicate dance of shadows and illumination. This phase, preceding the complete cessation of menstrual cycles, introduces itself with nuanced changes that might elude the untrained eye, signaling the body's gradual pivot towards a new state of equilibrium. Menstrual irregularity emerges as the harbinger of this transition, manifesting in cycles that stretch and contract unpredictably, as if the body itself is testing the waters of change. The flow, too, varies from its known patterns, alternating between scant and abundant, an echo of the hormonal fluctuations stirring beneath the surface.

The duration of Perimenopause, much like its symptoms, refuses to adhere to a prescribed timeline, spanning a spectrum from a few brief years to a decade or more. This variability underscores the profoundly personal nature of the process, a journey that unfolds at its own pace, guided by the body's intrinsic rhythm. Symptoms may ebb and flow with the tides of hormonal shifts, presenting a moving target for those seeking to understand and manage this phase of life.

Among the early signs, sleep disturbances frequently surface, casting a shadow overnights that once promised rest. Women might find themselves wading through the mists of insomnia, or jolted awake by night sweats, the remnants of dreams evaporating as quickly as the peace that accompanied them. Urinary issues, too, mark their territory in this landscape of change, with urgency and frequency becoming unwelcome companions, a reminder of the body's evolving narrative. Changes in libido weave through this tapestry, a nuanced thread reflecting the complex interplay of hormones, emotions, and physical well-being.

In preparing for the transition that Perimenopause heralds, a mosaic of lifestyle adjustments emerges as a canvas for self-care and resilience. Nutrition claims its place at the forefront, serving as a cornerstone for maintaining balance and vitality. A diet rich in whole foods, fibers, and phytonutrients becomes the daily bread, fueling the body with the elements needed to navigate the fluctuations of hormones and energy. Exercise, too, stands as a pillar of support, its value extending beyond physical health to encompass emotional and cognitive well-being. Participating in consistent activities such as brisk walks or morning yoga sessions cultivates endurance, strength, and a sense of stability amid transitions.

Parallel to these adjustments, consultations with healthcare providers bridge the gap between experience and understanding, offering insights tailored to individual needs and conditions. These conversations serve as lighthouses, guiding women through the fog of uncertainty that can accompany Perimenopause. They offer a space for questions to be voiced and fears to be acknowledged, for the narrative of menopause to be reframed not as an ending but as a continuum of women's health. In this dialogue, the options for managing symptoms are laid bare, from hormonal therapies that whisper to the body in its own language to alternative remedies that draw on the healing wisdom of nature.

In navigating the early signs of Perimenopause, women learn to attune themselves to the nuances of their bodies, interpreting its signals with a newfound literacy. This attunement fosters a partnership with the self, a collaboration honing the body's wisdom and capacity for adaptation. It cultivates a landscape where change is with curiosity rather than fear, where each symptom and shift becomes a thread in the larger tapestry of life. Through this lens, Perimenopause reveals itself not as a disruption but as a dialogue, an invitation to engage with the body in its journey through the seasons of womanhood.

As the early signs of Perimenopause unfold, they beckon women to embrace this phase with awareness and compassion, to navigate the transitions with an anchor of knowledge and a sail of resilience. In doing so, they chart a course through the waters of change, guided by the stars of self-care and supported by the currents of community and connection.

1.5 When It's Not Just Menopause: Other Causes of Similar Symptoms

Navigating the waters of midlife changes requires a map that distinguishes the landmarks of menopause from other territories marked by health conditions with similar signposts. The landscape is often misty, with symptoms such as fatigue, mood swings, and sleep disturbances masquerading as mere travelers from the land of menopause when, in reality, they hail from different provinces altogether. This misattribution can lead a woman to misunderstand her body's signals, over-looking the true origins of her experiences.

The body speaks a language nuanced with subtleties, where a symptom like fatigue can be a whisper from an underactive thyroid, a condition known as hypothyroidism, rather than a shout from the hormonal shifts of menopause. Similarly, the valleys of mood swings and depression may owe their depths not to the ebbing estrogen but to clinical depression, a condition that requires its own form of navigation. Heart palpitations often waved away as a common menopausal symptom, can sometimes signal cardiovascular issues, requiring immediate attention rather than dismissal under the broad umbrella of menopause.

In this complex terrain, medical evaluation is crucial as it guides women to seek clarity about the origins of their symptoms. A thorough health assessment, including blood tests and evaluations, becomes critical in charting the correct course. This evaluation aims to illuminate the landscape, distinguishing between symptoms rooted in menopause and those signaling other health conditions such as thyroid disorders, depression, or even heart disease. This distinction is crucial, for the path of treatment diverges significantly based on the underlying cause, each condition demanding its own tailored approach.

The potential for misdiagnosis looms as a shadow over this journey, a reminder of the importance of advocating one's health. It is a call to engage with healthcare providers, question, seek second opinions when necessary, and insist on comprehensive evaluations. This advocacy is not born from a place of doubt towards medical professionals but from an understanding that the body's whispers can sometimes be misinterpreted, leading to treatments that walk down one path. At the same time, the real issue lies in another. Advocacy becomes a bridge to the correct diagnosis, ensuring that the treatment plan illuminates the true nature of one's symptoms.

The differentiation between hormonal imbalance and other medical conditions is akin to distinguishing between two dialects of the same language. It requires attentiveness to the body's signals, an openness to exploring various possibilities, and a partnership with healthcare professionals who can interpret these signals within the broader context of one's health. For instance, while hot flashes and night sweats might wave the flag of menopause, they can also be emissaries from the realm of endocrine disorders or infections. Weight changes, too, often attributed to the hormonal shifts of menopause, can signal thyroid issues or metabolic syndrome.

This nuanced understanding invites a holistic approach to symptom management that considers the entirety of a woman's health landscape. It encourages a dialogue between patient and practitioner, a collaborative effort to trace symptoms back to their roots, whether they be nestled in the soil of menopause or branching out from other conditions. This dialogue is done with respect for the complexity of the female body and an acknowledgment that its messages are multifaceted and require careful interpretation.

In this quest for clarity, detailed health histories become paramount. These histories, narratives of one's body through time, offer clues that can direct the investigative process. When listened to attentively, they are stories that can reveal patterns and anomalies pointing toward the trustworthy source of symptoms. Coupled with diagnostic testing, these histories form the foundation of a targeted approach to symptom management that addresses the root cause rather than merely silencing the symptoms.

As women navigate this landscape, they become cartographers of their own health, mapping the contours of their symptoms, and distinguishing between the provinces of menopause and other health conditions. This mapping is not a solitary task but a collaborative endeavor involving healthcare providers, families, and the broader community. It is a journey marked by questions, learning, and commitment to understanding the body's language in all its complexity.

In the realm of women's health, where symptoms often cross borders between different conditions, the ability to differentiate is a powerful tool. It empowers women to seek targeted, effective treatments, advocate their health confidently, and navigate the midlife transition with an informed understanding of their body's messages. This differentiation ensures that the journey through menopause and beyond is marked not by confusion or misdiagnosis but by clarity, health, and well-being.

2 | Nourishing Balance Through Menopause

Imagine your body as a finely tuned instrument, each part contributing to the harmony of the whole. Menopause, then, becomes a time when the strings might feel a bit out of tune. The food and nutrients we introduce into our system act as the tuner, realigning our body's harmony. This chapter delves into the symphony of diet and nutritional strategies that support the body through menopause, focusing on the significance of certain nutrients, foods to embrace or avoid, the role of phytoestrogens, and maintaining a healthy weight.

2.1 Diet and Nutritional Strategies

Nutritional Needs During Menopause

The body's nutritional demands shift with menopause. Calcium and vitamin D become paramount for maintaining bone density, countering the elevated risk of osteoporosis. The daily ballet of nutrients doesn't stop there; magnesium for muscle function, B vitamins for energy, and omega-3 fatty acids for heart health play leading roles. Embracing a diet rich in these nutrients supports not just the physical but also the emotional and cognitive realms affected by menopause.

Foods to Favor and Avoid

Just as a musician selects the right notes to bring a piece to life, choosing the right foods can alleviate menopausal symptoms. Leafy greens, rich in calcium and magnesium, and fatty fish, a source of omega-3s, should take center stage in meals. On the flip side, spicy foods, caffeine, and alcohol might need to exit stage left for some, as they can exacerbate hot flashes and disrupt sleep patterns. Identifying personal triggers can be as enlightening as tuning into a favorite melody, and recognizing which foods harmonize with your body's current needs.

Role of Dietary Phytoestrogens

Phytoestrogens, naturally occurring plant compounds that mimic estrogen, play a nuanced role in the menopausal diet. Found in soy products, flaxseeds, and legumes, they can offer a gentle nudge towards hormonal balance. Yet, like a complex piece of music, the body's response to phytoestrogens varies from one individual to another. Some may find relief in symptoms, while others notice no change. The key lies in listening to your body's response and adjusting your diet accordingly.

Weight Management

Gaining weight during menopause is like adding unwanted dissonance to a melody. Changes in metabolism and hormone levels play a part, but they're not the sole conductors of this shift. Addressing weight gain involves a symphony of actions: mindful eating, focusing on nutrient-dense foods, and embracing regular physical activity. Imagine redesigning your plate to include a colorful array of vegetables, lean proteins, and whole grains, each bite contributing to a composition that supports a healthy weight and overall well-being.

Strategies for Incorporating Menopause-Friendly Foods

Creating a menopause-friendly diet doesn't require completely overhauling your eating habits overnight. It's about making incremental changes, like introducing one new vegetable or whole grain into your weekly meals. Consider the Mediterranean diet as a template, renowned for its balance of healthy fats, proteins, and abundant fruits and vegetables.

Consider gradual reductions rather than abrupt cuts for those accustomed to morning coffee or spicy food. Swap out your morning caffeine for green tea, which offers a gentler lift and is rich in antioxidants. Experiment with herbs and spices like turmeric or ginger to add flavor without the heat that can trigger hot flashes.

Incorporating these strategies into daily life doesn't demand perfection; it's about progress and tuning into what makes your body feel its best. Remember, the goal is harmony, not a strict adherence to rules that feel discordant with your lifestyle.

Visual Element: The Menopause Plate

A visual guide, "The Menopause Plate," illustrates an ideal balance of foods to support health during menopause. This infographic divides a plate into sections allocated for vegetables, fruits, whole grains, lean proteins, and healthy fats, with annotations on the benefits of each and suggestions for daily servings. It serves as a quick reference to visualizing balanced meals, making dietary adjustments more approachable and less overwhelming.

Interactive Element: Dietary Symphonies

A series of interactive prompts encourages readers to craft their "Dietary Symphony." This exercise invites you to list your favorite foods from each nutrient group essential during menopause, then mix and match them to create a week's worth of balanced meals. The aim is to see dietary planning as a creative and enjoyable process, akin to composing a piece of music that resonates with your body's needs.

By embracing these dietary strategies, we can support our bodies through the menopausal transition, finding balance and well-being in the process. It's about nourishing ourselves with care, tuning into our nutritional needs, and making mindful choices that bring harmony to our health.

2.2 Exercise as a Keystone Habit

Within the tapestry of the menopausal transition, threads of physical activity weave resilience, strength, and equilibrium into the fabric of daily living. The commitment to regular exercise emerges as a pivotal anchor, offering a counterbalance to the fluctuations of menopause, a period often marked by physical and emotional upheavals. The act of moving one's body transcends mere physical benefits, extending its reach into the realms of emotional stability, mental clarity, and a profound connection with one's bodily existence.

The Benefits of Regular Exercise

Physical activity, in its myriad forms, casts a wide net of benefits that touch upon the various symptoms and challenges of menopause. Hot flashes, those unpredictable surges of warmth, find a surprising adversary in the steadiness of exercise-induced thermoregulation. Bones, potentially weakened by the hormonal shifts of menopause, are fortified through weight-bearing activities, their density preserved or even enhanced against the tide of osteoporosis. Muscle mass, prone to decline with age, finds renewal in the challenge of resistance training, maintaining functional strength, and metabolic vigor. Beyond the tangible, the nebulous clouds of menopausal mood swings dissipate under the influence of endorphins released during physical exertion, offering solace in the storm.

Recommended Types of Exercise

The symphony of menopausal management calls for a harmonious blend of cardiovascular, strength, flexibility, and balance exercises, each contributing a unique tone to the overall composition. Cardiovascular activities, from brisk walks to cycling, ignite the heart's fire, improving endurance and heart health while serving as a crucible for burning away stress. Strength training, whether through bodyweight exercises or using weights, builds a fortress around bones and muscles, protecting against the siege of age and hormonal decline. Flexibility exercises, found in the gentle flow of yoga or the deliberate stretches of a cool-down, offer solace to joints and muscles, keeping the body limber and responsive. Balance exercises, often overlooked, play a crucial role in preventing falls, a concern heightened by the potential for brittle bones.

Starting an Exercise Routine

The initiation into regular exercise does not demand a leap but rather a series of small, intentional steps. For those previously less active, the beginning might look like a daily walk, its distance gradually expanding as comfort and capability grow. It's not the magnitude of the activity but the consistency that forges the path to benefits. Setting realistic goals, starting with ten minutes of daily activity and increasing incrementally, creates a scaffold of achievable milestones. Integrating physical activity into daily rituals—taking the stairs instead of the elevator, a stand-up meeting instead of sitting—seamlessly weaves exercise into the fabric of everyday life.

Overcoming Barriers to Exercise

The path to regular physical activity often involves tangible and intangible obstacles. Time, or the perceived lack thereof, looms large, its specter casting a shadow over intentions. Here, the reevaluation of priorities, the carving out of time from less essential activities, becomes an act of self-care, an investment in future well-being. Fickle and fleeting motivation often requires external bolstering—finding an exercise buddy, joining a class, or setting up a reward system can transform an activity from a chore into a cherished part of the day.

For some, physical limitations or discomfort pose a significant hurdle, demanding adaptations or modifications to exercise plans. Consulting with a physical therapist or a fitness professional knowledgeable about menopause can tailor activities to individual capabilities, ensuring safety and effectiveness. The exploration of low-impact exercises such as swimming, cycling, or pilates offers avenues for movement that are gentler on joints while still providing substantial benefits.

In this changing landscape, physical activity is a beacon of empowerment—a means through which women can reclaim agency over their bodies and well-being during menopause. The initiation and maintenance of an exercise routine tailored to individual needs and circumstances offer not just a mitigation of symptoms but a celebration of capability, resilience, and the joy of movement. Through the deliberate act of exercising, women forge a path through menopause marked by strength, balance, and a deep, abiding connection to the trans- formative power of their own bodies.

2.3 Sleep Quality and Menopause

In the menopause narrative, the plot thickens when night falls; sleep, once a trusted ally, morphs into a capricious companion. The hormonal upheaval characteristic of this phase disrupts the circadian rhythms, making insomnia and night sweats frequent plot twists in the otherwise tranquil nights. Progesterone, known for its soothing qualities, diminishes, leaving a void where sleep struggles to find its foothold. Estrogen's retreat further complicates this landscape, exacerbating temperature regulation issues that manifest as night sweats, pulling women from the depths of slumber into wakefulness.

Addressing these nocturnal disturbances requires a strategy as multifaceted as the symptoms themselves. The cornerstone of this approach lies in sleep hygiene, a series of practices designed to make sleep more reliable. Central to this is creating a sleep sanctuary, a bedroom environment optimized for comfort and relaxation. This means cooling the room to counteract the warmth of night sweats, choosing bedding that wicks away moisture, and investing in a mattress and pillows that support the body in its quest for rest. Light, too, plays a crucial role; its natural and artificial regulation cues the body's internal clock, signaling when it's time to sleep and wake. Dimming lights as evening falls and limiting screen time before bed can help reinforce the body's circadian rhythm, nudging it gently toward rest.

Establishing a bedtime routine is a prologue to sleep, signaling to the mind and body that it's time to wind down. Include practices such as gentle stretching to release physical tension, a warm bath scented with lavender to soothe the senses, or a period of reading that allows thoughts to drift away from the day's stressors. Consistency in this routine, both in activities and timing, strengthens the body's association between these practices and sleep, smoothing the transition from wakefulness to sleep.

In the realm of supplements and aids, melatonin emerges as a character of interest, and its role in regulating sleep cycles is well-documented. However, approaching its introduction into the body's ecosystem should be done cautiously, with mindfulness of the delicate balance involved. Herbal remedies, too, hold a place in this narrative, with valerian root and chamomile among the cast of herbs traditionally used to invite sleep. Yet, here lies a plot twist: the efficacy and safety of these aids are not universally guaranteed, and their interaction with the body's unique chemistry is unpredictable. Thus, the exploration of supplements and herbal remedies unfolds best under the guidance of a knowledgeable healthcare provider, ensuring that this path toward sleep remains intact.

Persistent sleep issues, those stubbornly resistant to sleep hygiene strategies and mindful supplementation, call for a deeper inquiry, a subplot that may require professional insight. This is where the narrative shifts from self-guided efforts to collaborative problem-solving with a healthcare provider. Sleep disturbances, persistent and pervasive, may hint at underlying conditions such as sleep apnea or anxiety disorders, requiring diagnostic exploration and targeted interventions. The dialogue with a healthcare professional opens a chapter of personalized strategies, potentially incorporating cognitive-behavioral therapy for insomnia (CBT-I) or exploring other medical or therapeutic avenues.

In this chapter of the menopause saga, the pursuit of sleep quality becomes an act of reclaiming the night, transforming it from a period of restlessness to one of restoration. The strategies outlined here and provided, such as improving sleep habits and seeking medical advice, offer a holistic approach to managing menopausal sleep challenges. Though at times arduous, this journey through the night holds the promise of dawn, a return to restful nights that support the body and mind through the transition of menopause.

2.4 Stress Management Techniques

In the labyrinth of menopause, stress acts not as a mere bystander but as an active participant, weaving its influence into the fabric of symptoms and experiences. This relation- ship between stress and menopause symptoms is neither straightforward nor benign; instead, it is a dynamic interplay where stress can intensify the common discomforts of menopause, further skewing hormonal equilibrium. Under- standing this link illuminates the necessity of cultivating stress mitigation practices, transforming them from optional activities into integral components of menopausal wellness.

The worsening of menopause symptoms under stress underscores the body's heightened sensitivity to external pressures during this transition. Hot flashes may surge in frequency and intensity, sleep might become even more elusive, and mood swings could swing with greater amplitude. This cascade of reactions is not a foregone conclusion but a call to action—an invitation to engage with stress management techniques that offer both immediate relief and long-term equilibrium.

Mindfulness and meditation emerge as powerful allies in this endeavor, offering a sanctuary of calm during hormonal storms. These practices root one in the present moment, curtailing the tendency to ruminate on past frustrations or future anxieties—a common catalyst for stress. By fostering an attentive engagement with the here and now, mindfulness and meditation can lower the volume of menopausal discomforts, providing a respite that rejuvenates both mind and body. The essence of these techniques lies not in their complexity but in their simplicity, accessible through guided sessions, digital applications, or even self-directed practices that weave mindfulness into daily routines.

Deep breathing exercises stand alongside as effective stress reducers, their efficacy rooted in the physiological response they elicit. By consciously slowing and deepening the breath, one can activate the body's relaxation response, counterbalancing the stress-induced fight-or-flight reaction. This shift from a state of heightened alertness to one of calm can dampen the impact of stress on menopause symptoms, acting as a buffer that softens the edges of hormonal fluctuations. Techniques like diaphragmatic breathing or the 4-7-8 method can serve as rapid stress-relief tools or as regular practices to establish a foundation of calmness.

Yoga, with its blend of physical postures, breath control, and meditation, offers a holistic approach to stress management during menopause. This ancient practice adapts to the practitioner's needs, accommodating varying levels of flexibility and strength. Yoga's benefits extend beyond the mat, influencing stress levels, mood, and even the physical manifestations of menopause, such as hot flashes and sleep disturbances. Regular engagement with yoga can thus serve as a comprehensive tool for navigating menopause with grace; its sequences are a physical metaphor for the balance one seeks during this period of change.

Creating a personalized stress-reduction plan transforms these techniques from isolated actions into a cohesive strategy tailored to one's lifestyle, preferences, and specific stressors. Such a plan might integrate daily mindfulness practice, weekly yoga sessions, and the use of deep breathing exercises as needed, alongside activities that inherently bring joy and relaxation. Whether it's immersing oneself in nature, engaging in creative pursuits, or cultivating social connections, these joy-filled activities enrich the stress-reduction plan, addressing the symptoms and the spirit.

Yet, there are moments when stress overwhelms, its waves crashing over the barriers one has carefully constructed. In these instances, the role of professional support becomes evident, serving as a lifeline back to equilibrium. Therapy or counseling, particularly cognitive-behavioral therapy (CBT), can unravel the knotted threads of stress, providing tools and insights that empower one to navigate through menopause's challenges with resilience. These professionals offer not just strategies for coping but a space for validation and under-standing, acknowledging the complex interplay between stress, menopause, and overall well-being.

The pursuit of stress management during menopause is not a solitary endeavor but a collective journey, supported by the wisdom of practices tested by time and the guidance of professionals attuned to the nuances of this life stage. In embracing these techniques, one seeks to diminish stress and cultivate a quality of life where balance, peace, and vitality are paramount. This approach to managing stress, rooted in both ancient practices and modern understandings, offers a pathway through menopause marked not by turmoil but by tranquility, transforming the experience into one of growth and profound personal discovery.

2.5 Holistic Approaches to Symptom Management

In the realm of menopause management, a tapestry of holistic and alternative remedies beckons with the promise of relief, weaving together ancient wisdom and contemporary practice. This section introduces a selection of non-medical approaches, including acupuncture, massage therapy, and the use of herbal supplements, each offering a pathway to symptom alleviation through means that extend beyond the conventional.

Acupuncture, with its roots burrowed deep in traditional Chinese medicine, stands as a beacon for those navigating the stormy seas of menopause. Tiny needles, when placed precisely along the body's meridians, are believed to restore the flow of qi, or vital energy, thereby encouraging balance and health. For women facing the fiery trial of hot flashes, acupuncture might offer solace, reducing both their intensity and frequency. Similarly, massage therapy, through the deliberate manipulation of body tissues, aims to release tension, improve circulation, and promote a sense of well-being that menopause often disrupts. The gentle pressure and rhythmic strokes of massage serve as a balm, soothing the aches and pains accompanying this transitional period.

It is turning to the realm of herbal supplements; a garden of possibilities unfolds, each plant offering its unique blend of compounds to address menopause symptoms. Black cohosh, known for its potential to ease hot flashes and night sweats, and St. John's Wort, often associated with relieving mild to moderate depression, are but two examples in a diverse botanical arsenal. Yet, it's crucial to tread this garden path with caution, as the efficacy and safety of herbal supplements can vary widely.

Amid these explorations, we must uphold the importance of actively evaluating the evidence. Scientific examination offers a perspective to evaluate the efficacy of holistic treatments, discerning between those supported by research and those relying solely on anecdotes. This discernment is vital, ensuring that women are empowered to make informed choices about their care. In this light, acupuncture's potential to mitigate hot flashes gains credence from clinical studies, while the use of certain herbal supplements finds support in systematic reviews. However, the evidence landscape is ever- evolving, necessitating ongoing inquiry and an open dialogue with healthcare professionals.

Crafting personalized treatment plans emerges as a corner-stone of holistic symptom management. Recognizing that menopause unfolds in a mosaic of patterns unique to each individual, tailoring approaches to fit one's specific needs and symptoms becomes a pivotal strategy. This customization considers not only the physical and emotional facets of menopause but also the lifestyle, preferences, and overall health of the woman at its center. It's a process that values the individual as a whole, seeking solutions that harmonize with her life rather than imposing a one-size-fits-all remedy.

Safety and interactions loom as critical considerations in this holistic approach, spotlighting the need for vigilance and partnership with healthcare providers. The terrain of alternative remedies, while rich with potential, is also fraught with the risk of adverse reactions and interactions, mainly when herbal supplements are introduced into a regimen that includes conventional medications. Consulting with health- care professionals ensures that these treatments do not veer into harmful territory, safeguarding against unintended consequences and guiding women toward options that enhance their well-being without compromise.

In the embrace of holistic and alternative remedies, women find a spectrum of options to navigate the multifaceted experience of menopause. From the ancient art of acupuncture to the healing touch of massage and the botanical diversity of herbal supplements, these approaches offer avenues to symptom relief that resonate with the body's natural rhythms. Yet, the journey through this landscape is one marked by careful consideration, informed by evidence, and tailored to the individual. It's a path that underscores the importance of partnership with healthcare professionals, ensuring that each step is grounded in safety and aligned with personal health goals.

In exploring holistic approaches to menopause management, the narrative weaves together the threads of ancient wisdom, contemporary practice, and the individual tapestry of symptoms and needs. It highlights the diversity of options available, the importance of evidence-based choices, and the imperative of personalized care plans. As we transition from this exploration, we carry forward the under- standing that managing menopause is not merely about alleviating symptoms but about nurturing well-being in its most total sense. This holistic perspective, embracing both alternative and conventional strategies, paves the way toward a balanced and healthful passage through menopause, opening the door to the next chapter of life with grace and empowerment.

Adaptogenic Herbs

Adaptogenic herbs are like nature's little helpers, working tirelessly behind the scenes to keep your body balanced and harmonious. They're like the superheroes of the plant world, swooping in to save the day when your body is under stress. Taking adaptogenic herbs is like having your plant allies by your side. They're always there to support you, no matter what life throws your way. Feeling anxious? Ashwagandha's got your back. Tired and run down? Rhodiola will give you a boost of energy. Dealing with hormonal imbalances? Maca's got you covered. And the best part is that adaptogenic herbs are natural and gentle on the body. They're like Mother Nature's little stress-busting, energy-boosting, mood- enhancing concoctions. So why not give them a try? You might find that your plant posse becomes your new best friend. You might even start talking to them like old pals and thanking them for their hard work and support. "Thanks, Rhodiola, you're a real lifesaver today!"

Of course, it's important to remember that adaptogenic herbs are just one part of a healthy lifestyle. They're not a magic cure-all, but they can help support your body and mind during stress and imbalance. As with any supplement, it's always a good idea to consult a healthcare provider before starting a new regimen. But with the proper guidance and approach, you might find that adaptogenic herbs become your new secret weapon for managing stress and improving your overall well-being.

Ashwagandha: This herb is known to help reduce stress and anxiety, improve sleep quality, and boost energy levels.

Rhodiola Rosea: Rhodiola can help improve mental clarity, reduce fatigue, and enhance physical performance.

Ginseng: Ginseng is known to boost energy, improve cognitive function, and enhance immune system function.

Maca: Maca is known to help balance hormones, improve fertility, and enhance libido.

Holy Basil· Holy basil, also known as tulsi, has been shown to help reduce stress and anxiety, improve digestion, and enhance immune system function.

Schisandra: Schisandra is known to help improve liver function, reduce oxidative stress, and enhance cognitive function.

Cordyceps: Cordyceps is known to help improve exercise performance, enhance immune system function, and reduce inflammation.

Reishi: Reishi is known to help reduce stress and anxiety, improve sleep quality, and enhance immune system function.

Eleuthero: Eleuthero, also known as Siberian ginseng, has been shown to help improve physical performance, reduce fatigue, and enhance immune system function. While adaptogenic herbs are known to have potential benefits, they are not a substitute for medical treatment or a healthy lifestyle.

Additionally, the appropriate dosage and possible interactions should always be discussed with a healthcare provider before taking supplements.

3 Embracing Emotional Equilibrium

Menopause, often cloaked in the guise of physical transformation, wields a less visible yet potent influence on the emotional landscape. Amidst the discourse on hot flashes and sleep disturbances lies a nuanced dialogue about the ebb and flow of emotions, an undercurrent that shapes the experience in profound yet often overlooked ways. This chapter delves into the intricacies of mood swings and emotional health during menopause, unraveling the threads that tether hormonal changes to emotional well-being and illuminating paths toward emotional regulation and resilience.

3.1 Understanding Mood Swings and Emotional Health

Hormonal Changes and Mood

The interplay between hormones and mood during menopause is akin to a dance, where estrogen and progesterone lead with steps that can either harmonize or disrupt the rhythm of emotional stability. As these hormones fluctuate, so does the brain's neurotransmitter activity, influencing mood, anxiety levels, and emotional reactivity, which vary among individuals. This biochemical choreography can result in mood swings that range from fleeting irritability to profound sadness, painting a complex emotional landscape for many.

Strategies for Emotional Regulation

In navigating this terrain, techniques for emotional regulation emerge as critical tools, offering ways to maintain balance amidst the hormonal storm. Mindfulness, for instance, anchors one in the present moment, creating space between emotional triggers and reactions. Through regular practice, mindfulness fosters a non-judgmental awareness of thoughts and feelings, allowing for a more measured response to emotional upheavals.

Cognitive Behavioral Therapy (CBT) offers another avenue for managing mood swings. It targets cognitive distortions that can amplify emotional responses. CBT equips individuals with strategies to challenge and reframe negative thought patterns, fostering a more adaptive and positive outlook on the menopausal transition and its impacts.

Emotional journaling provides a conduit for expression, offering a private space to explore thoughts and feelings freely. This practice not only aids in processing emotions but also in identifying patterns and triggers of mood swings, providing insights that can inform more mindful responses to emotional shifts.

The Importance of Self-Awareness

Cultivating self-awareness stands at the core of emotional well-being during menopause, demanding an attuned and compassionate attention to one's internal states. For instance, recognizing the signs of an impending mood swing can empower one to employ techniques like deep breathing or a mindful walk, intercepting the emotional spiral before it escalates. This self-awareness extends to understanding the multifaceted nature of menopause, acknowledging that emotional fluctuations are a natural and valid aspect of the experience.

Seeking Professional Help

There comes a moment when the waves of emotion might overwhelm, signaling a need for professional support. Mental health professionals specialize in navigating the complexities of mood and emotional health, offering a lifeline to those finding it challenging to manage independently. Whether through therapy, counseling, or possibly medication, professional intervention can provide a structured approach to emotional regulation tailored to the individual's unique circumstances and needs.

Interactive Element: Mood Mapping Exercise

A mood mapping exercise invites readers to chart their emotional landscape over a week. By recording moments of heightened emotion alongside the context in which they occur, individuals can uncover patterns and triggers of mood swings.

This exercise, structured as a simple chart with prompts for time, emotion, context, and response, serves as a practical tool for increasing self-awareness and identifying strategies for emotional regulation.

Menopause, while often framed within the context of physical health, significantly influences the emotional domain. Understanding the relationship between hormonal changes and mood swings, coupled with strategies for emotional regulation, self-awareness, and professional support, equips individuals to navigate this aspect of menopause with resilience and grace. Through the practices of mindfulness, CBT, and emotional journaling, along with the guidance of mental health professionals, it becomes possible to maintain emotional equilibrium, embracing the menopausal transition not as a period of loss but as an opportunity for growth and self-discovery.

3.2 The Role of Mental Health Support

In the tapestry of emotional well-being during menopause, threads of mental health support are interwoven with resilience, understanding, and healing. This support, multifaceted in its nature, encompasses therapy, counseling, and the solidarity found within support groups. Each strand offers its unique sustenance, addressing the emotional and psychological upheavals accompanying this period of transformation.

The Types of Mental Health Support

The landscape of mental health support is rich and varied, offering solace and strategies through therapy. This process facilitates self-discovery and coping mechanisms under the guidance of a trained professional. By sharing this therapeutic goal, counseling often provides emotional support and problem-solving strategies in a more immediate, sometimes shorter-term context. Whether convened in person or virtually, support groups present a platform for shared experiences, creating a community of empathy, understanding, and collective wisdom. These groups can be specific to menopause or, more broadly, focus on women's health, yet all strive to diminish the isolation accompanying this phase of life.

The Benefits of Professional Guidance

Engagement with mental health professionals unveils a spectrum of benefits, illuminating strategies and tools that ease the navigation through menopause-related challenges. These experts, whether therapists, counselors, or psychologists, bring to light coping mechanisms tailored to the individual's emotional landscape, fostering resilience against the tides of change. The guidance provided extends beyond mere symptom management, delving into the roots of emotional turmoil to foster a deeper understanding of oneself. This professional support acts as a catalyst for growth, encouraging the exploration of personal strengths and vulnerabilities with compassion and insight.

Accessing Resources

The quest for mental health resources, crucial to this journey, requires both awareness and action. Local health centers and hospitals often serve as starting points, offering referrals to therapists and counselors specializing in women's health and menopause. The digital realm expands these horizons, hosting directories of mental health professionals alongside virtual support groups and forums. These online platforms break down geographical barriers, rendering support accessible from the comfort of one's home. Furthermore, professional associations related to psychology and women's health frequently provide resources and connections to specialists in this field, ensuring that individuals can find the support that resonates with their specific needs.

Normalizing Mental Health Care

Amidst the evolution of societal perspectives on health, the normalization of seeking mental health support during menopause emerges as a vital shift. This transformation in collective consciousness challenges the stigmas that have long shrouded mental health care in the shadows of judgment and misunderstanding. Advocacy for this cause, both within communities and through media platforms, champions the message that mental well-being is integral to overall health. By fostering open dialogues about the emotional complexities of menopause, the cloak of invisibility that has historically enveloped this subject begins to lift.

This openness not only empowers individuals to seek the support they need but also fosters a culture of empathy and understanding that acknowledges the emotional dimensions of menopause as deserving of care and attention.

In the realm of menopause, where physical symptoms have often usurped the spotlight, the role of mental health support stands as a testament to the inseparability of mind and body. Therapy, counseling, and support groups offer beacons of hope and understanding, guiding individuals through the emotional undercurrents of this life stage. Pursuing such support, grounded in recognition of its value and the normalization of its necessity, weaves a more substantial fabric of emotional well-being. Professional guidance, accessible resources, and societal advocacy empower individuals to navigate the emotional intricacies of menopause with strength, clarity, and a sense of connectedness. This approach, holistic in its embrace of mental health care, illuminates a path toward resilience and renewal, where emotional equilibrium is not just a distant hope but a tangible reality.

3.3 Cultivating Self-Compassion and Acceptance

In the throes of menopause, the path to self-compassion emerges as a beacon, illuminating the way toward inner peace and acceptance of oneself. This pivotal concept, self-compassion, embodies the practice of greeting one's experiences, especially those tinged with discomfort or perceived inadequacy, with kindness and understanding. It acknowledges one's humanity, recognizing that the physical and emotional oscillations experienced are not aberrations but facets of a natural process.

Self-compassion becomes particularly poignant as bodies morph in ways that society, with its rigid beauty standards, might not always celebrate. Amidst this, the internal narrative can skew towards self-critique, a harsh dialogue that magnifies every hot flash and night sweat into a symbol of decline. Here, the cultivation of self-compassion acts as an antidote, a soothing balm that transforms internal discourse into one of nurturing and empathy. It encourages recognizing these changes not as failings but as markers of a significant life transition, deserving of care rather than condemnation.

The practices for building self-acceptance are manifold, each serving as a step toward reconfiguring one's self-image into one that radiates positivity. Visualization exercises, for instance, invite reimagining one's body as a vessel of strength and resilience. Through guided imagery, individuals can foster a connection with their physical selves that is rooted in gratitude for the body's enduring support, rather than in scrutiny of its changes. Affirmation practices further this journey, with repeated, positive declarations about one's worth and capabilities cementing a foundation of self-belief and acceptance. When woven into the fabric of daily life, these affirmations gradually shift perceptions from critical to compassionate.

The specter of self-criticism often looms large during menopause, its presence a testament to ingrained patterns of negative self-talk. With its ceaseless commentary on every perceived flaw, this internal critic requires a confrontation with gentleness and determination. The strategy involves:

- ➲ Actively monitoring thoughts.
- ➲ Catching the critic in the act.
- ➲ Challenging its assertions with evidence of one's worth, resilience, and achievements.

Though requiring persistence, this mental recalibration diminishes the power of self-criticism, substituting it with a narrative that advocates self-compassion and realistic self-assessment.

Self-care rituals underscore the importance of self-compassion, embodying the physical manifestation of this internal attitude. These rituals, tailored to personal interests and needs, range from the simplicity of a skincare routine that honors the body to indulgence in activities that nourish the soul, such as reading, gardening, or creative pursuits. Each act of self-care, no matter how mundane it may appear, is a declaration of self-worth, a reaffirmation of the commitment to treat oneself with the same kindness one would extend to a cherished friend. Through regular engagement in these practices, self-care becomes a cornerstone of daily life, each ritual a thread in the tapestry of self-compassion.

Nutrition and physical activity, too, play critical roles in cultivating self-compassion. The conscious choice to fuel the body with foods that enhance vitality and to engage in movement that celebrates its capacity rather than punishing it for its changes is an act of reverence. It acknowledges the body's needs and commits to meeting them with respect, fostering a relationship with oneself based on nurturing rather than on deprivation or criticism.

In this landscape, we cannot overstate the importance of social connections and meaningful relationships. Surrounding oneself with individuals who uplift and affirm can mirror back the self-compassion one is striving to internalize. Conversations that validate and empathize with the menopausal experience reinforce the normalcy and universality of this transition, dissolving the isolation that might otherwise cloud one's perception of self-worth.

Mindful engagement with hobbies or activities that spark joy is a conduit for self-compassion. Each pursuit reminds us of the facets of identity that persist beyond menopause. This engagement enriches the present moment and cements a sense of self that is multifaceted and resilient, capable of growth and discovery irrespective of age or life stage.

The narrative of self-compassion and acceptance in the context of menopause is one of transformation, a journey from self-critique to self-care, from resistance to embrace. It is a path marked by the understanding that the fluctuations of the body and mind are not detriments but aspects of a phase rich with potential for introspection, growth, and renewal. Through the practices of visualization, affirmation, challenging negative self-talk, and indulging in self-care rituals, the journey toward self-compassion unfolds, each step a movement towards an embrace of the self that is as nurturing as it is liberating. In this embrace lies the power to navigate menopause not as a period of loss but as an opportunity for profound self-discovery and acceptance, a chapter in the larger story of one's life where the protagonist emerges not only unscathed but enriched, empowered, and enveloped in self-compassion.

3.4 Building a Supportive Community

In the domain of menopause, the quest for solace and understanding often leads to the creation or discovery of supportive communities. These enclaves, whether formed in the physical realm or cultivated in the digital expanse, function as sanctuaries where individuals share experiences, exchange advice, and dispel the sense of expertise solitude like mist dissipating under the morning sun.

Finding Support Groups

The initial step towards weaving this vital social fabric involves the meticulous search for existing groups focused on menopause and women's health. Libraries, community centers, and health clinics frequently serve as nodes in this network, offering information on local meetings where conversations about menopause flow freely. The digital land- scape expands this search exponentially, with forums, social media platforms, and dedicated websites hosting vibrant communities that span the globe. Here, the barriers of geography and time dissolve, allowing for exchanging stories, remedies, and support at any hour.

Navigating through these options requires a discerning eye that seeks spaces where positivity, respect, and genuine support are the pillars. Find a group where the collective voice uplifts, questions receive insight and empathy, and the diversity of menopausal experiences.

Benefits of Shared Experiences

The act of sharing one's journey through menopause with others traversing similar paths casts a light on the commonality of experiences, despite the variability of symptoms and coping strategies. This communion brings with it a profound sense of relief, breaking the shackles of isolation that can often accompany this phase. The stories shared within these groups paint a picture of resilience, a mosaic of individual battles fought with courage and, sometimes, a touch of humor. It's in the laughter shared over a hot flash anecdote or the collective nodding at the mention of sleepless nights that a powerful realization dawns—no one is alone in this.

The exchange of knowledge within these groups often acts as a beacon, guiding members through the fog of misinformation and toward evidence-based strategies for managing symptoms. Here, personal anecdotes of what worked and what didn't become invaluable gems of wisdom, each contributing to the collective knowledge repository. Furthermore, the emotional support that flows freely in these gatherings offers a cushion against the impact of menopause on mental and emotional well-being, providing a sense of belonging that bolsters the spirit.

Creating Your Own Support Network

For some, the perfect fit still needs to be discovered among the existing groups. In such instances, the spark to form a new group ignites a venture that, while daunting, holds the potential to fulfill not only one's own needs but those of others searching for their tribe. Initiating such a group starts with identifying the core focus—emotional support, sharing natural remedies, or navigating healthcare options. With a clear purpose, outreach can begin, tapping into personal networks, community boards, and online platforms to gather like-minded individuals.

Setting the tone for open, respectful, and positive interaction from the outset lays the foundation for a supportive environment. Establishing regular meetings, whether in person or online, creates a rhythm and a predictable sanctuary where members can share and learn. As the group evolves, its members become the architects of its culture, each contributing to the growth and direction of the community.

Support from Healthcare Providers

Integral to the fabric of support is the relationship with healthcare providers, a partnership that extends the network beyond the peer level to incorporate professional guidance. These professionals, be they doctors, nurses, or specialists in women's health, offer a wealth of knowledge and experience, providing a medical perspective that complements the anecdotal wisdom of support groups.

Engaging healthcare providers in conversations about menopause, armed with questions and a desire to understand, transforms these interactions into opportunities for more profound insight. A dialogue fosters concerns and options, and we can make decisions collaboratively. This partnership doesn't replace the peer support network but enriches it, ensuring the group's shared information is balanced with professional advice.

In this collective endeavor, the support network becomes a tapestry, interwoven with the threads of personal experiences, professional insights, and the unconditional support of peers. It's a living entity, evolving with the needs and contributions of its members, offering a haven where the journey through menopause is not a solitary trek but a shared voyage. Through the act of building and nurturing these communities, individuals find not only support and understanding but also the powerful affirmation that in the face of menopause, they stand together, united in strength and resilience.

3.5 Communication Strategies with Family and Partners

Navigating the fluctuating waters of menopause requires not only an internal compass but also the guidance and understanding of those closest to us. In sharing our experiences with family and partners, we find solace and a shared language for the myriad changes unfolding. Opening this dialogue, however, demands a delicate balance, a nuanced approach that fosters understanding without seeding alienation.

Opening the Dialogue

Initiating conversations about menopause with those we hold dear is akin to planting a garden together, which requires both tenderness and patience. It begins with choosing a moment of calm, a space free from the distractions and pressures of daily life where thoughts and feelings can flow unimpeded. In these shared moments, we can unfold the menopause narrative, introducing it not as a series of medical symptoms but as a personal tide of change, rich with emotional and physical nuances. The aim here is to invite our loved ones into our experience, offering them a window into the complexities of our internal world.

Educating Loved Ones

We are with the understanding that knowledge is the bedrock of empathy; providing our family and partners with resources and information about menopause becomes a critical step in bridging the divide of experience. This education goes beyond mere facts, delving into the personal impact of menopausal changes and highlighting how they affect the individual and the fabric of our relationships. Books, articles, and reputable online resources can serve as shared points of reference, springboards for deeper discussions that illuminate the multifaceted nature of menopause. The goal is to transform the unknown into the familiar, dismantling myths and misconceptions to build a foundation of shared under- standing.

Setting Boundaries and Needs

In articulating the contours of our needs and establishing clear boundaries, we create a map for our loved ones to follow that guides them in how to support us best. This process is less about erecting barriers and more about delineating the landscape of our emotional and physical well-being. It involves candidly disclosing what we find helpful versus what might exacerbate our discomfort, inviting our partners and family to be allies in navigating menopause. The specificity of this communication ensures that support is not a broad gesture cast into the void but a targeted embrace that meets us where we are.

Coping Strategies for Partners

Equipping our partners with coping strategies is an act of collective resilience, a way to arm our shared ship against the storms of menopause. It's about acknowledging that while the experience is intensely personal, its ripples touch those around us, often leaving them feeling powerless or adrift. By sharing strategies that delineate how they can support us—through understanding, patience, or practical help—we empower them to be active participants in this phase of life. This empowerment might manifest in simple acts, like taking over specific responsibilities during times of acute discomfort or learning the subtle art of providing space when needed. In these acts, support finds its most accurate expression, in the willingness to navigate the complexities of menopause as a united front.

In weaving together these communication strategies, we forge connections that transcend the barriers of experience, crafting a shared narrative that encompasses not just the challenges of menopause but the strength of vulnerability. By opening the dialogue, educating our loved ones, setting clear boundaries, and equipping our partners with coping strategies, we ensure that the journey through menopause is not a solitary path but a shared voyage. In the confluence of these communication streams, understanding deepens, relationships fortify, and the menopausal transition becomes a bridge to greater intimacy and connection.

As this chapter draws to a close, the essence of our exploration into communication strategies with family and partners crystallizes into a simple truth: menopause, in all its complexity, offers an opportunity to deepen the bonds we share with those closest to us. Through open dialogue, education, clear communication of needs, and mutual support, we not only navigate the challenges of menopause but also cultivate relationships that are richer, more understanding, and resilient. These strategies, rooted in honesty, empathy, and shared learning, pave the way for a journey through menopause that is less about enduring and more about evolving together.

4 | The Mosaic of Menopause

Menopause, often misconstrued as a monochromatic phase of life, reveals itself as a vibrant mosaic of experiences, each tile a story, a shade, a texture that contributes to the collective masterpiece. Within this mosaic, individual stories of menopause, distinct yet interconnected, weave a tapestry of shared humanity. These narratives, rich in diversity and depth, serve not only as a mirror reflecting the myriad ways in which menopause touches lives but also as a window into the soul of womanhood in its most transformative stage.

4.1 Diverse Experiences of Menopause

The Collection of Stories

A tapestry gains its beauty from the variety of threads it encompasses, and similarly, the menopause experience draws its essence from the multitude of individual stories it encompasses. Whether it unfolds in a metropolitan city's bustling streets or the rural landscape's tranquility, each narrative adds a unique hue to the collective understanding of menopause. These stories span the spectrum from those who navigate this transition with minimal disruption to their daily life to those for whom menopause is a tumultuous sea of physical and emotional upheaval.

Universal Themes

Despite the diversity, specific threads run daily through the fabric of menopause stories. Themes of renewal, resilience, and rebirth emerge, painting a picture of menopause not as an end but as a beginning—a second spring. These universal themes bind the individual narratives, creating a shared language of experience and understanding. They remind us that beneath the surface differences, the core of the menopause experience resonates with a familiar chord of human emotion and physicality.

Cultural Perspectives

The lens of culture shapes the perception and experience of menopause, coloring it with societal norms, traditions, and attitudes. In some cultures, menopause is undoubtedly as a rite of passage, a welcome transition into a respected phase of wisdom and freedom. In others, it is veiled in silence, its symptoms and significance shrouded in a cloak of invisibility. Exploring these cultural narratives offers a kaleidoscopic view of menopause, highlighting how societal context influences the individual experience and the communal discourse around this phase of life.

Empowerment through Sharing

The act of sharing menopause stories is an act of empowerment, a declaration that these experiences matter and that they deserve a voice in the broader narrative of women's health. In the sharing, there is a dismantling of stigma, a breaking of silences that have long surrounded this transition. For many, hearing the stories of others becomes a beacon of hope, a reassurance that they are not alone in their experience. It fosters a sense of community and solidarity, offering strength to those who might otherwise feel isolated in their journey.

Visual Element: The Menopause Mosaic

An infographic entitled "The Menopause Mosaic" visually represents the diversity of menopause experiences across different cultures, ages, and lifestyles. This mosaic, composed of individual tiles that depict unique stories, collectively forms a vibrant image that celebrates the spectrum of menopause. Accompanying each tile is a brief narrative or quote, capturing the story's essence. This visual element high- lights the diversity and common threads woven through the menopause experience, offering viewers a multifaceted understanding of this phase of life.

Interactive Element: Mapping Your Menopause Story

A guided journaling exercise, "Mapping Your Menopause Story," invites readers to contribute their own thread to the tapestry. This exercise provides prompts that encourage reflection on the physical, emotional, and cultural dimensions of their menopause experience. Questions guide users to explore how their cultural background has influenced their perception of menopause, what universal themes they find in their own stories, and how the act of sharing or listening to menopause stories has impacted them. This interactive element fosters a deeper personal understanding and enriches the collective narrative by adding more voices to the chorus of menopause experiences.

This chapter uncovers the richness of this phase of life by delving into the diverse experiences of menopause, from collecting individual stories to exploring cultural perspectives. It celebrates the universal themes that unite these experiences while honoring the differences that make each story unique. Through sharing and listening, women find empowerment, drawing strength from the mosaic of menopause that reflects not just a transition but a transformation.

4.2 Lessons Learned from Long-Term Menopause Survivors

Wisdom grows from the soil of experience, nurtured by the trials and triumphs of those who have navigated the terrain of menopause with resilience. These sages, women who have traversed the ebbs and flows of hormonal shifts, offer beacons of insight, illuminating the path for others still finding their way. Their voices, rich with the gravitas of lived experience, echo with advice and strategies that transcend the passage of time, offering a compass to guide us through the disruption of transition.

These survivors share a repository of knowledge that isn't captured in the pages of medical textbooks but resides in the fabric of their daily lives. They speak of the alchemy of patience and persistence, of learning to listen to the whispers and roars of their bodies with an attuned ear. It is a dialogue, they remind us, that does not happen overnight but develops with the passage of moons and the turning of seasons. Among their most cherished insights is the art of adaptation—finding solace in the cooling embrace of a fan during a hot flash or the comfort of layered clothing that can be shed light on at a moment's notice. They advocate the sanctity of sleep, recommending dark, cool rooms free of electronic distractions and perhaps the inclusion of gentle, natural sleep aids like lavender or chamomile.

Yet, beyond the practicalities, these veterans of change speak to the heart of the menopause experience—the interior landscape marked by shifting emotions and the quest for equilibrium. They counsel the cultivation of practices that anchor the spirit, whether through meditation that grounds and centers or through hobbies that distract and delight. They remind us that the tempest of emotions is not an enemy to be defeated but a wave to be ridden gracefully, acknowledging its presence while seeking the shore of calm on the other side.

One of the most resonant pieces of wisdom they share is perspective transformation. They view menopause not as a diminishment but an evolution that opens new vistas of self-discovery and growth. This shift in viewpoint is not about denying the challenges but embracing them as opportunities to learn, adapt, and thrive. It reframes the menopause experience as a passage to a new chapter of life, rich with possibility, rather than merely an ending.

And what of life beyond the symptomatic storm of menopause? Here, the survivors offer a glimpse and a clear vista of a landscape where calm has returned, the body has found its new rhythm, and life unfolds with a richness informed by the journey. They speak of a renewed sense of self, of energies redirected from the management of symptoms to the pursuit of passions long deferred. This phase, they assure, is marked not by loss but by liberation—the freedom from menstrual cycles, the unshackling from the fear of pregnancy, and the embrace of a body that has weathered change and emerged resilient.

In this realm beyond symptoms, the survivors underscore the significance of nurturing the body and spirit with continued attention to nutrition and physical activity, tailored now not to the management of menopause but to the celebration of vitality. They advocate maintaining the social connections forged in the crucible of transition, for these bonds, tempered by shared experience, hold a depth and resilience that enrich life in profound ways.

The tapestry of advice and insight these long-term survivors share weaves a narrative of hope and resilience. It offers a roadmap through the shifting terrain of menopause, marked by practical strategies for managing symptoms and enriched by a perspective that sees beyond the immediate to the promise of what lies ahead. Their wisdom, born of experience, stands as a testament to the capacity for adaptation, growth, and renewal that defines not just the menopause transition but the journey of life itself.

4.3 Men Supporting Women Through Menopause

In the intricate dance of relationships, the onset and progression of menopause introduce a rhythm that demands patience and a profound depth of understanding from partners. Stories of men who have journeyed through these experiences with their partners shed light on paths guided by empathy, mindfulness, and a steadfast dedication to providing support. Their diverse stories converge on the common ground of love and respect, offering invaluable insights into how men can stand as pillars of strength and understanding during this transformative period.

Stories from Supportive Partners

Within these shared experiences, a mosaic of support strategies emerges, each tailored to the unique dynamics of the relationship and the individual needs of the woman under-going menopause. One narrative recounts the journey of a husband who sought to educate himself on the physiological and emotional shifts of menopause, arming himself with knowledge to understand better the storms his wife faced. Another speaks of a partner who, recognizing the unpredictability of mood swings, cultivated an environment of open communication and patience, ensuring their home remained a sanctuary of peace and understanding.

These tales, while varied, underscore a common theme: the pivotal role of active engagement and empathy. Partners who navigate this phase successfully complete do so not by standing on the sidelines but by immersing themselves in the experience alongside their loved ones, armed with an open heart and a willingness to adapt.

Understanding and Empathy

The cornerstone of support during menopause rests on a foundation of understanding and empathy. It requires an acknowledgment that while the menopause experience is deeply personal, its repercussions ripple through the fabric of the relationship. Partners adept at providing support strive to perceive the world through the lens of their loved ones, recognizing that empathy is not about fixing problems but about sharing their burden.

In this context, empathy manifests in myriad ways, from the simple act of listening without judgment to the more tangible steps of adjusting the household's routine to accommodate the fluctuating needs of a partner undergoing menopause. It might mean embracing cooler room temperatures for comfort or encouraging and participating in activities that alleviate stress and promote well-being.

Advice for Men

For men seeking to support their partners through menopause, the advice distilled from the experiences of others who have walked this path is both practical and profound. Begin with education, they suggest, for under- standing demystifies menopause, transforming it from a feared unknown into a phase of life to navigate with compassion. Communicate in moments of calm and during turmoil, ensuring that the lines of dialogue remain open and free from judgment.

Men are encouraged to cultivate patience, recognizing that the journey through menopause is not linear but marked by peaks and valleys. This patience also extends to themselves, acknowledging that there will be moments of frustration and helplessness, but that perseverance and empathy can weather these storms.

Flexibility, too, is crucial. The ability to adapt to a partner's changing needs and moods during menopause speaks volumes of a man's commitment to the relationship. It might mean taking on additional responsibilities within the house- hold or finding new ways to connect and express affection that acknowledges the physical and emotional changes occurring.

The Impact on Relationships

Navigating menopause together, with understanding and empathy, can fortify a relationship's bonds, embedding layers of depth and resilience previously untapped. The shared experience of menopause, with its challenges and triumphs, serves as a crucible that strains and ultimately strengthens the relationship.

Partners who approach this phase as a team find that their relationship evolves, characterized by a deeper appreciation for the nuances of communication, the importance of empathy, and the value of shared vulnerability. This evolution reflects not just the survival of menopause but also the thriving, where the relationship becomes a testament to the power of partnership in facing life's transitions.

In this shared journey, the relationship itself and emerges transformed, characterized by a richness that comes only from weathering storms together. It becomes a relationship marked not just by love but by a profound understanding and respect for the journey each has undertaken, both individually and together.

Through the narratives of men who have supported their partners through menopause, through the advice distilled from their experiences, and through the reflection on the impact of this journey on relationships, a blueprint emerges. It is a blueprint not for navigating menopause with ease but for doing so with grace, understanding, and an unwavering commitment to supporting and ensuring that the journey through menopause, while challenging, becomes a shared voyage towards a deeper, more resilient connection.

4.4 The Role of Online Communities in Menopause Support

In an era where digital connectivity weaves into the fabric of daily existence, the quest for understanding and companionship amidst the waves of menopause finds a harbor in the vast sea of the internet. Online forums, social media groups, and digital communities dedicated to menopause are sanctuaries where voices, silenced or diminished in the physical realm, amplify with resonance and reach. These digital congregations serve not merely as repositories of shared knowledge but as the very embodiment of solidarity and support across the ether.

Finding Online Support

Navigating the labyrinthine expanse of the internet to uncover these havens of support necessitates a discerning eye and an open heart. With their algorithmic precision, search engines become the initial scouts, leading seekers to forums and websites where conversations about menopause flourish. Social media platforms, too, offer gateways to groups and pages dedicated to the menopausal experience, each click a step closer to a community that understands, empathizes, and embraces. Yet, the true essence of finding support online lies not in the mere act of joining these digital spaces but in the active engagement with them. Participation, whether through sharing one's own narrative or responding to another's, transforms passive observation into a dynamic exchange of wisdom, comfort, and camaraderie.

Virtual Friendships and Connections

Within these online communities, threads of connection weave into the tapestry of virtual friendships, bonds formed in the crucible of shared experience. Stories of such connections abound, tales of individuals who, though separated by continents and cultures, find kinship in their mutual traverse through menopause. These friendships, nurtured through messages, comments, and shared stories, blossom into significant sources of support and understanding. They stand as a testament to the power of digital communities to transcend the physical barriers that often constrain our social interactions, offering a profound and far-reaching sense of belonging.

Navigating Online Information

Yet, the abundance of information characterizing these online spaces demands a critical lens through which to sift the valuable from the vacuous. While a cornerstone of internet culture, the democratization of knowledge also paves the way for misinformation to proliferate amidst the genuine wisdom. Thus, the savvy navigator of online menopause support learns to question, verify, compare sources, and seek evidence-based advice. This discernment ensures that the guidance gleaned from these digital interactions enriches rather than misleads, grounding decisions in reliable and relevant information.

Privacy and Safety Online

Amidst the openness that characterizes online discussions, preserving privacy and safety is paramount. Engaging in conversations about menopause, while liberating, also exposes individuals to the vast, anonymous audience of the internet. Caution becomes the watchword, guiding the amount and nature of personal information shared in these digital forums. Many learn to navigate this balance through using pseudonyms or participation in closed groups, strategies that allow for openness without sacrificing personal privacy. Moreover, the vigilance against potential online predators or scams underscores the importance of maintaining a guardedness even while seeking connection and support.

Navigating the balance between transparency and prudence defines the quest for menopause support online. It is a journey marked by the discovery of kindred spirits, the acquisition of knowledge, and the cultivation of a supportive network that spans the globe. In these online communities, individuals find not just information but a sense of identity within the shared narratives of menopause, a reassurance that they are neither alone nor without resources in this transition. The digital age, with all its complexities, offers a unique opportunity to connect, learn, and grow within the context of menopause, reshaping the experience from one of isolation to one of communal traverse and mutual uplift.

4.5 Creating Your Own Menopause Story

In the canvas of existence, every individual paints their narrative with strokes broad and fine, colors vivid and subdued, creating a masterpiece uniquely theirs. Within the realm of menopause, the act of documenting one's personal evolution through this transformative phase becomes a powerful medium of expression and introspection. Engaging in journaling, blogging, or other avenues of storytelling offers a conduit for the raw, unfiltered essence of this experience to flow, capturing the nuances of change in a medium that endures.

The potency of storytelling lies in its capacity to serve as both a mirror and a window. It reflects the depth of one's internal landscape while offering a glimpse into how menopause reshapes life's contours. This duality is not merely an exercise in self-expression but a profound journey into self-awareness. Through the written word, emotions find clarity, confusion finds direction, and the chaos of transformation finds order. The narrative becomes a tangible thread connecting past, present, and future, weaving a coherent story from the disparate elements of experience.

Reflecting on and writing about one's journey through menopause does more than chronicle a series of events; it facilitates a process of emotional digestion. The act of translating thoughts and feelings into words demands a level of engagement with one's inner world that is both illuminating and cathartic. It requires pausing to listen to the whispers of change, acknowledge the shouts of frustration, and honor the silence of acceptance. This introspection fosters a deeper comprehension of how menopause is not merely a physical transition but a pivotal point of psychological and emotional growth.

Sharing one's menopause story, whether with a close circle of friends or a broader audience through blogging or social media, extends an invitation for connection and community. It transforms personal narrative into a beacon for others navigating similar waters, offering solace in shared experience and strength in collective wisdom. The decision to make one's journey public is a testament to the power of vulnerability as a catalyst for bonding and understanding. It underscores the notion that while menopause is a universal phenomenon, its impact is rich in the diversity of individual stories.

Moreover, the legacy of support that these narratives create cannot be understated. They become part of a larger tapestry of knowledge and empathy, a resource for future generations seeking guidance and solace as they approach or journey through menopause. The stories left behind are not merely accounts of personal experience, but lanterns lighting the path for others, illuminating the challenges, triumphs, and transformative potential of menopause. They stand as evidence that while the physical aspects of this phase may fade with time, the emotional and psychological growth it engenders leaves an indelible mark on the fabric of one's being.

In sharing these narratives, the storyteller not only contributes to the collective understanding of menopause but also to the dismantling of taboos that have long shrouded this transition in secrecy and shame. It is an act of reclamation, asserting the significance of menopause as a vital chapter in the story of womanhood, deserving of recognition and respect. Through the act of storytelling, menopause is reframed from a period of loss to one of gain, a gain in knowledge, self-awareness, and the depth of connection to oneself and others.

As we weave the final threads of this chapter, it becomes clear that the act of documenting and sharing one's menopause story is a profound tool for navigation and growth. It is a practice that transcends the individual, touching the lives of others and contributing to a broader narrative of empowerment and understanding. The narratives we share and exchange contribute to a mosaic, each one a fragment of the broader portrait of menopause, capturing its beauty, intricacy, and profound transformative potential. Turning the page, we step into the next chapter, enriched by the knowledge and insights gained, ready to explore new dimensions of this journey with openness and curiosity.

Women Want to Hear Your Story!

Around Half the World's Population Will Experience Menopause...Yet We Still Can't Share Our Individual Experiences!

> *"If men went through menopause, we'd know everything about it, but we still don't even know if we should be taking hormones,"*
>
> — *Joycelyn Elders*

This statement isn't meant to offend men, many of whom are highly supportive. At the same time, we also know quite a few who have a cold yet insist they are dying of the flu. It's not easy for them to understand the true struggles women go through during menopause.

But this isn't their fault. It's not from a lack of willingness on their part, but rather a societal issue where, despite the prevalence of menopause, women aren't encouraged to talk about it. This means that both genders are often left in the dark.

The words "no period" and "hot flashes" are the most familiar images of menopause, but this ignores the other 32 major symptoms women can go through.

Each experience is unique, and women who are going through or about to undergo this significant life change deserve to hear these unique perspectives.

And, whether it's your boss, partner, or even your son, the men in your life deserve this information, too.

There is a simple but incredibly powerful way to break the silence surrounding menopause, and it doesn't involve shouting your story from the rooftops!

Women want to hear your story and know what strategies and techniques have helped you manage your symptoms and lead a positive, happier life. Your review on Amazon is the perfect way to reach out to these women...and the men who want to support them!

It only takes a few minutes but those few minutes will make a huge difference to someone who is in the same place you were a few chapters ago. Thank you so much, and on that note, let's get back to your personal experience and learn how to get the most out of the menopausal years!

Scan the QR code below

SCAN ME

5 Navigating the Maze of Menopause Information

In a world awash with information, discerning the wheat from the chaff becomes an art form, especially when it pertains to navigating menopause. The swirling in the vast ocean of data, myths cozy up alongside facts, personal anecdotes masquerade as universal truths, and sales pitches often overshadow science. The quest for reliable menopause resources mirrors a trek through an intricate maze, where each turn and decision point demands scrutiny and a keen sense of direction.

5.1 Finding Reliable Menopause Resources

Wisdom grows from the soil of experience, nurtured by the trials and triumphs of those who have navigated the terrain of menopause with resilience. These sages, women who have traversed the ebbs and flows of hormonal shifts, offer beacons of insight, illuminating the path for others still finding their way. Their voices, rich with the gravitas of lived experience, echo with advice and strategies that transcend the mere passage of time, offering a compass to guide us through the disruption of transition.

These survivors share a repository of knowledge that isn't captured in the pages of medical textbooks but resides in the fabric of their daily lives. They speak of the alchemy of patience and persistence, of learning to listen to the whispers and roars of their bodies with an attuned ear. It is a dialogue, they remind us, that does not happen overnight but develops with the passage of moons and the turning of seasons. Among their most cherished insights is the art of adaptation

—finding solace in the cooling embrace of a fan during a hot flash or the comfort of layered clothing that can be shed light on at a moment's notice. They advocate the sanctity of sleep, recommending dark, cool rooms free of electronic distractions, and perhaps the inclusion of gentle, natural sleep aids like lavender or chamomile.

Yet, beyond the practicalities, these veterans of change speak to the heart of the menopause experience—the interior landscape marked by shifting emotions and the quest for equilibrium. They counsel the cultivation of practices that anchor the spirit, whether through meditation that grounds and centers or through hobbies that distract and delight. They remind us that the tempest of emotions is not an enemy to be defeated but a wave to ride gracefully, acknowledging its presence while seeking the shore of calm on the other side.

One of the most resonant pieces of wisdom they share is perspective transformation. They view menopause as not a diminishment but an evolution that opens new vistas of self-discovery and growth. This shift in viewpoint is not about denying the challenges but about embracing them as opportunities to learn, adapt, and thrive. It reframes the menopause experience as a passage to a new chapter of life, rich with possibility, rather than merely an ending.

And what of life beyond the symptomatic storm of menopause? Here, the survivors offer a glimpse and a clear vista of a landscape where calm has returned, the body has found its new rhythm, and life unfolds with a richness informed by the journey. They speak of a renewed sense of self, of energies redirected from the management of symptoms to the pursuit of passions long deferred. This phase, they assure, is marked not by loss but by liberation—the freedom from menstrual cycles, the unshackling from the fear of pregnancy, and the embrace of a body that has weathered change and emerged resilient.

Identifying Credible Sources

Like a seasoned chef selects only the freshest ingredients for a gourmet meal, finding trustworthy information on menopause requires a discerning eye for quality. Peer- reviewed studies stand out as the gold standard, with rigorous scrutiny by experts ensuring a level of reliability unmatched by anecdotal evidence. With their commitment to evidence- based practice, reputable health organizations serve as beacons guiding seekers through the fog of misinformation. The North American

Menopause Society (NAMS) and the Women's Health Initiative (WHI) exemplify such sources, their publications and guidelines offering a solid foundation for understanding menopause.

Leveraging Digital Resources

The digital age unfurls a tapestry of resources at our fingertips, from scholarly articles accessed through academic databases to forums where healthcare professionals dispense advice. Websites dedicated to women's health, such as WebMD and Mayo Clinic, provide a wealth of information, from symptom management to the latest research findings. Apps designed to track menopause symptoms can also offer personalized insights, making the abstract deeply personal.

Utilizing Libraries and Bookstores

Local libraries and bookstores offer a treasure trove of knowledge for those who prefer the tactile sensation of flipping through pages. Menopause, once a topic shrouded in whispers, now claims its rightful place on shelves, with titles ranging from scientifically dense tomes to light-hearted memoirs. Visiting the library might reveal "The Menopause Manifesto" by Dr. Jen Gunter. This book blends medical expertise with feminist insight, offering a comprehensive look at menopause within the larger context of women's health.

Healthcare Professionals as Resources

Yet, sometimes, the most reliable resource for all the written words and digital bytes is a conversation with a healthcare provider. These professionals, from family physicians to gynecologists specializing in menopause management, offer personalized advice and a human touch. They can clarify doubts, debunk myths, and guide decisions on treatment options, making them invaluable allies in the quest for information.

Visual Element: The Menopause Information Maze

An infographic, "The Menopause Information Maze," visually represents the journey to find reliable menopause resources. It illustrates paths leading to various sources, such as scholarly articles, reputable health organizations, digital apps, and healthcare professionals, with caution signs marking dubious information sources. This visual guide simplifies the search for quality information. It highlights common pitfalls to avoid, making the quest for knowledge more manageable.

Interactive Element: Menopause Resource Checklist

A downloadable checklist, "Menopause Resource Checklist," aids readers in evaluating the reliability of information sources. It includes criteria such as author credentials, citation of scientific studies, endorsement by health organizations, and the presence of peer reviews. This tool empowers readers to become savvy consumers of menopause information, equipping them with the skills to discern quality resources in their exploration.

In this era of information overload, navigating the maze of menopause resources demands both critical thinking and a proactive approach. Individuals can arm themselves with accurate and applicable knowledge by identifying credible sources, leveraging both digital and traditional mediums, and engaging with healthcare professionals. Though fraught with challenges, this journey ultimately leads to a place of understanding and empowerment, where decisions about menopause management rest on solid ground.

5.2 The Importance of Ongoing Education

In the landscape of menopause management, the terrain is ever-shifting, shaped by the winds of new research and the tides of evolving understanding. The imperative for those navigating this phase is not merely to amass a static pool of knowledge but to engage in the continuous pursuit of learning, ensuring that the strategies and decisions that guide them remain rooted in the most current science and practices. This commitment to ongoing education opens a gateway to empowerment, allowing individuals to advocate their health with both confidence and flexibility.

Staying Updated with Research

The realm of menopause research is dynamic, where discoveries and insights emerge at a pace that demands attentive- ness. For those seeking to manage their menopausal journey with informed precision, keeping abreast of these developments is not optional but essential. Academic journals and publications dedicated to women's health serve as vital conduits for the latest findings, offering a glimpse into the scientific community's ongoing dialogue about menopause. Engaging with this material allows individuals to sift through the layers of emerging data, distinguishing between fleeting trends and substantive advances in understanding and treatment. It is a practice that transforms passive healthcare recipients into proactive participants, armed with questions and a keen eye for how new research might refine or redefine their approach to menopause management.

Educational Workshops and Seminars

Beyond the solitary act of reading and research lies the interactive world of workshops and seminars, platforms where knowledge is transmitted and shared. These gatherings, whether held in person or in the increasingly accessible digital space, offer a unique blend of education and community. Participants find themselves in the company of experts and peers, creating an environment ripe for exchanging ideas, experiences, and strategies. The value of these events extends beyond the information presented; they foster connections and networks that can support and enrich one's menopause journey. Experts leading these sessions provide nuanced insights into the practical application of research findings, bridging the gap between scientific theory and day-to-day management. For many, these workshops and seminars become a cornerstone of their ongoing education, a place to learn, question, challenge, and deepen their understanding.

Subscribing to Health Newsletters

In the digital age, the flow of information is relentless, a constant stream that can overwhelm as much as it informs. Subscribing to newsletters from trusted medical institutions or societies dedicated to menopause offers a way to filter this stream, curating a flow of relevant, reliable information directly to one's inbox. These newsletters, often penned by experts in the field, distill the essence of new research, policy changes, and emerging trends into digestible summaries. They serve as a beacon for busy individuals, highlighting significant developments without the need to navigate the vast ocean of available data. This targeted approach to staying informed ensures that crucial insights and recommendations are noticed, integrating seamlessly into the rhythm of daily life.

The Role of Patient Advocacy Groups

At the confluence of personal experience and collective action lie patient advocacy groups and organizations that do more than educate—they empower. These groups not only disseminate information but also champion the rights and needs of those navigating menopause. Membership in such groups offers access to a wealth of resources, from educational materials developed with the input of healthcare professionals to advocacy toolkits that equip individuals to engage in policy-making processes. The role of these organizations extends into the realm of research as well, often facilitating or funding studies that address their members' specific concerns and needs. Engaging with patient advocacy groups transforms the individual quest for knowledge into a shared endeavor, where education is a tool for personal management and a means to effect broader change. Through these groups, individuals gain more than just access to information. Still, it is a voice in the dialogue about menopause, contributing to a future where a diverse array informs management strategies of experiences and needs.

In this pursuit of ongoing education, the journey through menopause becomes one not of static endurance but of dynamic engagement. Staying updated with research ensures that management strategies evolve with the science. At the same time, participation in workshops and seminars fosters a community of learning and support. Subscribing to health newsletters offers a curated approach to staying informed, and involvement with patient advocacy groups empowers individuals to advocate themselves and the broader community. This approach to menopause, rooted in continual learning and proactive engagement, ensures that the management of this phase is as informed, current, and effective as possible, reflecting not just the state of the science but the lived experiences of those it seeks to serve.

5.3 Advocating Menopause Awareness

In the tapestry of modern discourse, threads of silence weave around the topic of menopause, often relegating it to the shadows of societal conversation. Yet, a revolution stirs, propelled by voices that refuse to be muted, advocating a world where menopause is not a whispered secret but a recognized and respected phase of life. This movement, fueled by the collective power of individuals and communities, seeks to dismantle the barriers of ignorance and stigma, advocating awareness, support, and policy change that uplift the experiences of menopausal women everywhere.

Raising Public Awareness

The digital age unfolds as a battleground for awareness, where social media platforms, blogs, and digital forums become the weapons of choice. Crafting content that resonates—be it through the raw honesty of personal blogs, the communal dialogue of social media posts, or the informative reach of online articles—serves as a clarion call to society. It beckons others to listen, learn, and engage with the realities of menopause, painting it not as an ailment but as an inherent part of the female existence. Organizing community events, whether virtual webinars or local gatherings, further amplifies this message, creating spaces where dialogue can flourish, free from the constraints of stigma or shame. These efforts, collectively, stitch a narrative of empowerment, weaving menopause into the fabric of public consciousness as a topic worthy of dialogue, understanding, and respect.

Lobbying for Policy Change

Beyond the realm of conversation lies the domain of action, where advocacy transcends words to manifest in the tangible change of policies and practices. The arena of workplace reform emerges as a critical battlefield, where advocates push for accommodations that acknowledge and support the needs of menopausal women. Lobbying for policies—such as flexible working arrangements, temperature control, and access to health resources—challenges employers to recognize menopause as a significant factor in the well-being of their workforce. Similarly, the call for healthcare reforms advocates for accessible, informed care that addresses menopause holistically, ensuring women receive the support they need without financial burden or discrimination. Engaging in letter-writing campaigns, participating in advocacy groups, and meeting with policymakers are actions that, when taken together, can shift the societal and institutional landscapes, embedding support for menopausal women into the very structures that govern daily life.

Participating in Research and Surveys

Knowledge is the foundation upon which effective advocacy rests, and participation in menopause-related research and surveys act as a keystone in this foundation. By contributing to studies that seek to understand the breadth and depth of menopause experiences, individuals offer invaluable data that can shape future understanding, treatment, and policy. Though perhaps small in isolation, these contributions aggregate into a powerful force for change, informing the scientific and medical communities about the realities of menopause on a granular level. Furthermore, surveys conducted by advocacy organizations or healthcare providers gather insights into the needs and preferences of menopausal women, guiding the development of services and resources that truly resonate with those they aim to serve. Participation in this research, therefore, is not merely an act of personal investment but a contribution to the collective well-being of all who navigate menopause.

Creating Support Networks

At the heart of advocacy lies the power of community, a force magnified by the creation and nurturance of support networks dedicated to menopause awareness and education. These networks, whether formal organizations or informal groups, serve as havens of information, empathy, and action. They provide a structure through which individuals can receive support and contribute to the broader movement of menopause advocacy. The act of forming such networks—or joining existing ones—fosters a sense of belonging among members, uniting them in their shared mission to elevate menopause to a place of recognition and respect within society. These networks disseminate knowledge, challenge misconceptions, and advocate systemic change through newsletters, educational programs, and advocacy initiatives. Moreover, they offer a blueprint for collaboration, demonstrating how collective action, rooted in shared experience and driven by a common goal, can dismantle the stigmas that have long silenced discussions around menopause.

In this concerted effort to advocate menopause awareness, the landscape of societal understanding and support trans- forms. Sharing stories, engaging in dialogue, lobbying for policy change, and participating in research have all taken strides towards a future where menopause is a natural, honored aspect of life. Through the creation and support of networks committed to this cause, the movement gains momentum, propelled by the strength of the community and the unyielding belief in the power of advocacy to enact change. In this journey, every voice that rises in support of menopause awareness weaves another thread into the fabric of societal consciousness, crafting a tapestry that, in its rich- ness and diversity, fully encompasses the breadth of the menopause experience.

5.4 Educating Men and Family Members

In the nuanced tapestry of familial dynamics, the thread of menopause weaves a complex pattern, often misunderstood or overlooked by those not directly experiencing its effects. Within this context, the act of conveying the breadth and depth of menopause's impact to family members and partners becomes not only an exercise in communication but a bridge to deeper connection and support. It requires a gentle hand to paint the landscape of menopause in hues that resonate with understanding and empathy, transforming potential divides into shared ground.

Effective Communication Strategies

The art of articulating the multifaceted experience of menopause to those closest to us demands both clarity and sensitivity. Initiating conversations with a mindset geared towards education rather than confrontation sets a foundation for openness. It is beneficial to frame these discussions around the tangible changes menopause introduces, not just physically but emotionally and psychologically, thus inviting our loved ones into a more profound comprehension of our experiences. A systematic approach, outlining specific symptoms or challenges alongside their impacts on daily life, can demystify menopause for family members and partners. It's akin to guiding them gently into a room they've never entered, illuminating corners and contours previously shad- owed or unseen.

Employing analogies that draw parallels between menopause and other life transitions experienced more universally can also bridge gaps in understanding. Such comparisons invite empathy by aligning the unfamiliar with the familiar, making the abstract concrete. Encouraging questions and discussions transforms these conversations into dialogues rather than monologues, fostering a dynamic exchange where curiosity leads to comprehension.

Educational Resources for Families

Curating a selection of resources tailored for those seeking to support their menopausal loved ones provides a scaffold for fostering comprehension. Books that approach the subject with a blend of humor and honesty, such as "The Madwoman in the Volvo: My Year of Raging Hormones" by Sandra Tsing Loh, can provide insights wrapped in relatability, making the topic approachable. Articles highlighting the latest research findings or personal essays reflecting the spectrum of menopause experiences broaden the perspective, presenting menopause not as a singular event but as a varied journey.

Online resources, particularly those hosted by reputable health organizations, offer accessible information designed to educate. Websites like the Mayo Clinic or The North American Menopause Society curate content that spans the scientific to the anecdotal, providing a well-rounded view of menopause. Directing family members and partners to these resources equips them with the knowledge that extends beyond the personal sharing, grounding their understanding in broader contexts.

Hosting an Educational Session

Convening an informal educational session at home, where family members and partners can delve into menopause's realities together, fosters a collective understanding. This gathering could involve watching documentaries that explore menopause, followed by discussions that allow for the expression of thoughts and feelings. It could also include reading segments from insightful books or articles and reflecting on them as a group. Such sessions, underscored by a spirit of learning and empathy, transform menopause from a topic skirted around to one engaged with openly and supportively.

Utilizing presentations or talks given by experts in the field, available through platforms like TED Talks or medical seminars online, introduces authoritative voices into the conversation, lending weight to the information shared. This collective educational endeavor, nestled within the comfort of a familiar environment, encourages a shared journey of understanding, dispelling myths, and fostering empathy.

The Role of Empathy

At the heart of these efforts lies the cultivation of empathy—a quality that binds the theoretical to the emotional, the factual to the felt. Family members and partners play a crucial role in nurturing empathy, allowing them to view the experience of menopause through a lens colored by compassion and understanding. It prompts a shift from the mere acknowledgment of the changes menopause brings to an active engagement with the support those changes necessitate.

Developing empathy might involve encouraging family members and partners to reflect on their physical or emotional challenges, drawing parallels to the unpredictability and intensity of menopause symptoms. It's about moving beyond sympathy, which observes from a distance, to empathy, which seeks to understand and share feelings. Such a shift deepens the emotional connections within the family or partnership. It creates a supportive environment where the individual navigating menopause feels seen, heard, and valued.

In the intricate dance of family dynamics, educating men and family members about menopause plays a pivotal role in harmonizing relationships during this transformative phase.

Through effective communication strategies, the selection and sharing of educational resources, the hosting of collaborative learning sessions, and the cultivation of empathy, the experience of menopause becomes a shared narrative. It transforms from a solitary journey into a communal voyage, marked by understanding, support, and a deepened bond that weathers the storms and celebrates the calm that follows.

5.5 The Role of Healthcare Professionals

Navigating the landscape of menopause with the support of healthcare professionals transforms an often solitary endeavor into a collaborative pursuit. This alliance, fortified by expertise and empathy, ensures that the voyage through menopause is informed and personalized, reflecting each individual's unique needs and concerns.

Building a Healthcare Team

The foundation of this partnership rests upon selecting and cultivating relationships with healthcare providers who bring not only a wealth of knowledge about menopause but also a genuine understanding of its multifaceted impact. A gynecologist, endocrinologist, or primary care physician interested in women's health can anchor this team, offering guidance grounded in the latest research and best practices. Yet, the composition of this team might extend beyond these traditional roles, incorporating nutritionists, physical therapists, or mental health professionals, each contributing a critical piece to the menopause management puzzle. Establishing this team requires proactive research, seeking recommendations from trusted sources, and scheduling introductory consultations to gauge the provider's approach to menopause care. It's a process akin to assembling a mosaic, where each professional represents a piece that, when combined, forms a complete picture of support.

Preparing for Medical Consultations

Preparation becomes pivotal to maximize the fruitfulness of interactions with this healthcare team. Before consultations, compiling a comprehensive list of symptoms, questions, and any current health strategies employed offers a clear agenda for discussion. This preparation might include maintaining a symptom diary, noting the frequency, intensity, and triggers of menopausal symptoms, and providing a tangible record that can inform treatment decisions. Articulating goals for the consultation and any concerns about treatment options or side effects ensures that the dialogue addresses the most pressing issues. This approach transforms the consultation into a dynamic exchange, where informed questions lead to insightful answers, and the path forward becomes a co- created strategy tailored to individual needs and preferences.

Advocating within the Healthcare System

Within the broader context of the healthcare system, advocating oneself emerges as a critical skill. This advocacy involves articulating one's needs clearly, requesting further clarification when explanations do not satisfy, and, if necessary, seeking second opinions to explore all available options. It's a stance that requires confidence, bolstered by the knowledge gained through ongoing education and the support of the healthcare team. At times, it might also involve challenging prevailing norms or recommendations, pushing for care that aligns with one's values and understanding of menopause. This active participation ensures that the healthcare system serves not as a maze but as a map, guiding individuals through menopause with clarity and purpose.

Navigating Insurance and Healthcare Policies

Understanding the intricacies of insurance coverage and healthcare policies is essential when navigating menopause. Policies regarding the coverage of hormone replacement therapy, alternative treatments, or consultations with specialists can significantly impact care decisions. Familiarizing oneself with the details of these policies, including any prerequisites for coverage or the process for filing appeals, equips individuals to make informed choices about their treatment plans. It might also involve direct negotiations with insurance providers, advocating the inclusion of specific therapies or treatments deemed necessary by the healthcare team. This navigation ensures that the journey through menopause is not hindered by bureaucratic obstacles but facilitated by a clear understanding of available resources.

As this exploration of the role of healthcare professionals in menopause management concludes, it underscores the importance of partnership, preparation, advocacy, and informed navigation within the healthcare landscape. This collaborative approach ensures that care is personalized, comprehensive, and aligned with the latest advancements in menopause research and treatment. It highlights the power of a well-constructed support system, where healthcare professionals guide and empower individuals to manage menopause with knowledge, confidence, and a sense of agency.

In the broader journey of menopause, the alliance with healthcare professionals stands as a testament to the strength of collaboration, ensuring that each step taken is informed, intentional, and tailored to the unique contours of individual experience. This chapter, in its exploration of building health-care teams, preparing for consultations, advocating within the system, and navigating insurance, offers a roadmap for engaging with healthcare professionals in a manner that respects the complexity and individuality of menopause. As we transition from this focus on the healthcare landscape, we carry forward the principles of informed partnership and proactive engagement. We are ready to explore new dimensions of managing menopause with an empowered and informed stance.

6 Implementing Change for a Better Menopause Experience

Menopause, with its unpredictable tides, calls for a detailed and flexible map that can adapt to the shifting sands beneath our feet. It's akin to preparing a garden for all seasons; understanding the soil, climate, and local wildlife is crucial to cultivating a space that thrives year-round. Similarly, personalizing your menopause plan requires an intimate understanding of your body's needs and responses, an ongoing dialogue between you, and the changing rhythms of your life.

6.1 Personalizing Your Menopause Plan

Assessing Individual Needs

The first step resembles a gardener testing the soil; it's about getting to the root of your menopausal symptoms, lifestyle nuances, and personal preferences. This process might unfold over a cup of morning tea, notebook in hand, as you jot down the symptoms that challenge you most, whether they be hot flashes interrupting your sleep or mood swings clouding your days. Reflect on your daily routines, dietary habits, and exercise patterns, noting any areas that might benefit from adjustment. This self-assessment is not a one-time task but an ongoing practice, much like a gardener who regularly checks their plants' health and soil quality.

Incorporating Holistic Approaches

With a clear understanding of your needs, the next step involves weaving holistic approaches into your plan. Imagine your menopause management as a garden where conventional medical treatments are just one plant species among many. Dietary changes, exercise routines, stress management techniques, and natural remedies are the companion plants, each contributing to the garden's overall health and balance. For instance, integrating phytoestrogen-rich foods like flaxseeds into your diet can be a natural way to balance hormones. At the same time, yoga or Tai Chi practices might serve as effective stress reducers, their gentle movements mirroring the ebb and flow of your breath and emotions.

Setting Realistic Goals

Establishing goals is like plotting a garden's layout before planting the first seed. It's about envisioning the garden you want to cultivate. However, it's vital to set goals that are as realistic as a gardener who understands that only some plants will thrive in its climate. Aim for gradual improvements and practice self-compassion, recognizing that growth takes time and patience. Your initial goal is to reduce the frequency of hot flashes through dietary adjustments or improve your sleep quality by establishing a calming bedtime routine. Whatever the goals, they should be markers on your path, flexible enough to adjust as you progress.

Reevaluating and Adjusting the Plan

As any seasoned gardener knows, a garden's needs change with the seasons, and what worked in spring might not suffice come fall. Likewise, your menopause management plan requires regular reevaluation and adjustment. This might mean revisiting your dietary choices if you notice certain foods trigger your symptoms or adjusting your exercise routine to suit your energy levels better. It's a process that might unfold during a quiet afternoon, with a garden or window view in sight, as you contemplate the adjustments needed to align your plan with your evolving needs.

Visual Element: The Menopause Management Map

An illustrated map serves as a visual guide to personalizing your menopause plan. It charts the terrain of menopause management, marking areas for self-assessment, holistic approaches, goal setting, and plan adjustment. Each map area is linked by paths that remind the reader of the journey's fluid nature, encouraging exploration and adaptation. This map, infused with botanical imagery, not only guides the reader through the steps of personalizing their menopause plan but also reinforces the concept of growth and change as natural, integral parts of the process.

Crafting a menopause plan that mirrors the intricacies of a well-tended garden shifts the emphasis from merely surviving menopause to thriving within it. It's a plan that grows with you, rooted in a deep understanding of your needs and blossoming into a holistic approach that nurtures your body, mind, and spirit. Through careful assessment, integrating varied strategies, realistic goal setting, and the flexibility to adjust, this plan becomes a living, breathing entity, as dynamic and resilient as the women it seeks to support.

6.2 Tracking Symptoms and Progress

In the realm of menopause management, the act of documenting fluctuations in symptoms and well-being serves as both a compass and a map, guiding adjustments to lifestyle and treatment with precision. The tools at our disposal, from analog journals to digital applications, enable a meticulous gathering of data, transforming subjective experiences into objective insights.

Utilizing Symptom Trackers

The digital age presents an arsenal of applications designed to monitor menopause symptoms, mood variations, and lifestyle factors, each functioning as a meticulous scribe of our daily experiences. These tools, ranging from simple trackers that record hot flash frequency to more sophisticated systems analyzing sleep patterns and diet, offer a panoramic view of our menopausal landscape. Custom alerts and reminders facilitate a consistent log of symptoms and encourage a proactive stance toward management. The data amassed over time reveals patterns and triggers, highlighting a correlation between sugar intake and mood swings or underscoring the impact of aerobic exercise on sleep quality.

Maintaining a Health Diary

The traditional health diary stands alongside the digital trackers, offering a canvas for a more nuanced narrative of our menopausal journey. This handwritten record, detailed in its scope, encompasses our days' physical symptoms, emotional currents, and dietary nuances. It invites reflection, urging us to note what we experience and how we respond physically and emotionally. The process of penning down these details fosters a mindfulness about our bodies and habits, illuminating the subtle shifts that might elude even the most attentive mind.

The diary becomes a repository of personal history, charting the ebbs and flows of menopause against the backdrop of our lives. It holds space for the fluctuations in our well-being, the efficacy of dietary adjustments, and the stabilizing power of physical activity, painting a holistic picture of our health that extends beyond mere symptomatology.

Analyzing Patterns and Trends

With the data from trackers and diaries in hand, the task then shifts to deciphering the narrative encoded within. This analysis, though meticulous, unveils the rhythms of our menopausal experience, identifying triggers that exacerbate symptoms and habits that offer relief. It might reveal, for instance, that the tendrils of stress weave through our days, tightening their grip on our well-being, or that the balm of meditation soothes the rough edges of our mood swings.

Patterns emerge from the fog of daily fluctuations, offering signposts for adjustment. A discernible link between caffeine consumption and sleep disturbances might prompt a reduction in coffee intake. At the same time, a clear correlation between journaling and the emotional equilibrium could encourage a commitment to daily reflection. This process of analysis, iterative in nature, demands patience and an open- ness to learning from the data we gather, allowing it to inform and refine our approach to menopause management.

Sharing Data with Healthcare Providers

When shared with healthcare providers, the insights gleaned from our symptom tracking and health diaries acquire additional value. This exchange, a confluence of personal observations and professional expertise, enhances the personalized nature of our menopause management. Healthcare professionals, equipped with a detailed account of our experience, can precisely tailor their advice and interventions, aligning treatment strategies with the nuances of our symptoms and lifestyle.

Sharing this data fosters a collaborative relationship with our providers, transforming the dynamic from passive receiving to active participation. It invites a dialogue where questions and concerns can be addressed with specificity, grounded in the reality of our daily experiences. Providers, in turn, gain a window into the complexities of our menopause journey, enabling them to offer solutions that resonate with our unique circumstances.

The data becomes a bridge in this shared space, connecting our lived experience with the broader landscape of menopause treatment and management. It underscores the importance of active engagement in our health care, empowering us to advocate our needs with evidence in hand. This partnership, informed by the rich tapestry of data we compile, ensures that our path through menopause is navigated with informed intention, personalized to our evolving needs, and responsive to the insights our own bodies provide.

6.3 Experimenting with Natural Remedies

In the realm of menopause management, the allure of natural remedies whispers of ancient wisdom and earth's bounty, promising relief in the folds of nature's apothecary. However, pursuing these remedies is not a mere amble through verdant fields of herbal promise but a deliberate, systematic quest for solutions that are at once effective and harmonious with our bodies' rhythms. This quest begins with the rigor of research. This fundamental step transforms the search from a foray into folklore to a science-informed exploration.

Researching Natural Remedies

Diving into the study of natural remedies demands a strategy that balances openness with skepticism and curiosity with caution. The vast sea of information available, from scholarly articles in databases like PubMed to discussions on dedicated forums, provides a fertile ground for discovery. Yet, it is critical to discern these waters, favoring sources that anchor their claims in scientific research over those buoyed by anecdotes alone. This research illuminates the landscape of options, from phytoestrogens found in soy and flaxseeds, known for their hormone-balancing potential, to black cohosh, a herb celebrated for its ability to temper hot flashes. Each remedy emerges under the scrutiny of science, revealing its mechanisms, benefits, and the depth of evidence supporting its use.

Starting with One Remedy at a Time

The initiation into natural remedies mirrors the careful cultivation of a garden, where introducing too many variables at once can obfuscate which plants thrive under specific conditions. Similarly, integrating one remedy at a time into your regimen allows for a clear assessment of its impact. This approach ensures that any changes in symptoms—be they improvements or adverse reactions—can be accurately attributed to the remedy in question. It is a practice that values precision over haste, allowing for the meticulous documentation of effects that inform whether a remedy deserves a place in your menopause management plan.

Monitoring and Documenting Effects

The diligent documentation of a remedy's impact is akin to keeping a detailed log of a scientific experiment. It involves noting the changes in the frequency and intensity of symptoms and any side effects that may arise. This record-keeping, whether in a digital app or a traditional journal, provides a timeline of experiences that can reveal patterns over time. Did the introduction of evening primrose oil coincide with a noticeable reduction in night sweats? Or did a regimen of ginseng bring with it unexpected irritability? These notes become invaluable data points, illuminating how each remedy interacts with your unique physiological landscape.

Consulting Healthcare Providers

Engaging in a dialogue with healthcare providers is a critical checkpoint in the experimentation with natural remedies. This conversation is a confluence of your lived experience and their medical expertise, a space where the personal insights gleaned from your documentation meet the broader perspective of scientific knowledge. Providers can offer guidance on the dosage, duration, and potential interactions of natural remedies, which is especially crucial for those navigating the complexities of multiple medications. This consultation ensures that your foray into natural remedies is grounded in safety and aligns it with the overarching strategy of your menopause management.

In this nuanced exploration of natural remedies, the journey is marked by the rigor of research, the strategy of incremental introduction, the discipline of monitoring, and the wisdom of professional consultation. Each step is taken with a mindfulness that respects both the potency of nature's offerings and the complexities of our bodies' responses. This approach, rooted in evidence and personalized care, transforms the quest for natural remedies into an informed exploration that honors the depth of traditional wisdom while anchoring firmly in today's science.

6.4 Navigating Medical Treatments

In the quest for equilibrium amidst the oscillations of menopause, the exploration of medical interventions serves as a critical chapter in the narrative of symptom management. This exploration is not a mere perusal of options laid out in the sterile confines of a doctor's office but a deep, discerning examination of treatments that span the conventional to the cutting edge. The landscape of medical treatments for menopause symptoms is as vast as it is varied, encompassing hormone replacement therapy (HRT), bioidentical hormones, and a plethora of alternative medications, each promising relief in the leaflets of their usage and the testimonies of those who've ventured before.

The initiation into this realm begins with an understanding that hormone replacement therapy, long regarded as the cornerstone of menopause management, offers a reprieve for many from the relentless waves of hot flashes, night sweats, and the myriad other symptoms that accompany this transition. Yet, HRT is neither a panacea nor a one-size-fits-all solution. Its efficacy and suitability are as individual as the patterns of a fingerprint, varying dramatically from one person to the next based on a complex interplay of health history, symptom severity, and personal health philosophies. Similarly, alternative medications, from the SSRIs used to temper mood swings to the blood pressure medications repurposed to quell hot flashes, present a tableau of options, each with its own profile of benefits and drawbacks.

HRT involves replacing the hormones that a woman's body is no longer producing in sufficient amounts during menopause. The two main hormones that are replaced are estrogen and progesterone.

It's important to note that HRT is not without risks and side effects, and it's not suitable for everyone. Women should discuss the potential benefits and risks of HRT with their healthcare provider to determine if it's the right option for them. HRT's type, dose, and duration depend on the individual's needs and medical history. Overall, HRT can be an effective treatment option for many women experiencing symptoms of menopause. By replacing the hormones, the body is no longer producing, HRT can help alleviate symptoms and improve the quality of LIFE.

Hot flashes and night sweats: HRT therapy can help regulate body temperature and reduce the frequency and severity of hot flashes and night sweats. It's like a personal air conditioner that can help keep you cool and comfortable, even in the hottest situations.

Vaginal health: HRT therapy can help maintain vaginal moisture and elasticity, preventing dryness, discomfort, and pain during sex. It's like a personal lubricant that can help keep things smooth and comfortable, even when the dry spell lasts a lifetime.

Bone health: HRT therapy can help maintain bone density and reduce the risk of osteoporosis and bone fractures. It's like a personal bodyguard who can help keep bones strong and healthy, even when gravity seems to be working against them.

Mental health: HRT therapy can help improve mood, reduce anxiety and depression, and enhance cognitive function It's like a personal cheerleader that can help keep your spirits high, even when life feels like a rollercoaster ride.

Cancer risk: HRT therapy can help reduce the risk of certain cancers, such as breast and endometrial cancer. It's like a personal bodyguard that can help keep you safe from harm, even when the odds seem stacked against you. It's important to remember that HRT is not without risks and side effects, and it's not suitable for everyone.

Testosterone therapy for women, while less commonly prescribed by conventional doctors, is sometimes offered by private healthcare providers specializing in hormone therapy. Testosterone is typically known as a male hormone. Still, it also plays a crucial role in women's health, contributing to energy levels, libido, muscle strength, and overall well-being. Women may experience low testosterone levels due to factors like aging, menopause, or certain medical conditions. Private doctors who offer testosterone therapy for women may consider it as part of a comprehensive approach to hormone optimization. Testosterone therapy in women can address symptoms such as low libido, fatigue, and decreased muscle mass. However, women need to undergo a thorough evaluation and discuss the risks and benefits of testosterone therapy with a qualified healthcare provider before starting treatment. Private doctors offering testosterone therapy for women aim to personalize treatment plans based on individual needs and health considerations. Regular monitoring and adjustments to the treatment regimen may be necessary to ensure its safety and effectiveness. Women seeking testosterone therapy should consult with a knowledgeable healthcare provider to explore this treatment option and determine if it aligns with their health goals and needs.

Bioidentical Hormone

Bioidentical hormones are a type of hormone therapy that uses hormones with a chemical structure identical to those naturally produced by the human body. These hormones are often derived from plant sources, such as soybeans or yams. They are used as an alternative to synthetic hormones. The idea behind bioidentical hormones is that they mimic the body's natural hormones more closely, potentially offering a more personalized and targeted approach to hormone therapy. It's like having a custom-made suit that fits you perfectly rather than a one-size-fits-all solution that might not be a perfect fit. Bioidentical hormones are commonly discussed in the context of natural or alternative treatments for hormone imbalances, such as those experienced during menopause. Menopause is a natural part of the aging process for women. Still, it can also bring about a host of uncomfortable symptoms, such as hot flashes, night sweats, mood swings, and vaginal dryness. HRT, including bioidentical hormones, is one way to alleviate these symptoms and improve quality of life. The beauty of bioidentical hormones is that they can be tailored to meet an individual's specific needs and preferences. A healthcare provider knowledgeable in bioidentical hormone therapy can work with a patient to determine the appropriate dosage and delivery method based on factors such as age, weight, medical history, and lifestyle. While bioidentical hormones have gained popularity in recent years, it's important to remember that they are not without risks and side effects. Some common side effects of HRT, including bioidentical hormones, include bloating, breast tenderness, headaches, and mood changes.

The process of evaluating the risks and benefits of these treatments unfolds through a dialogue that extends beyond the exchange of medical facts to encompass personal values, fears, and aspirations. It is a dialogue that demands transparency from healthcare providers about the potential side effects of HRT, such as increased risks of certain cancers or cardiovascular events, weighed against the relief it may offer from the immediate discomforts of menopause. Likewise, discussing alternative medications necessitates candidly examining efficacy, side effects, and how these treatments align with one's health journey. This evaluation is not a static process but an ongoing conversation that evolves with emerging research, health status shifts, and personal comfort with risk changes.

Personalizing treatment plans in this context becomes an art form that requires a keen sensitivity to the nuances of one's body and life circumstances. It is about crafting a regimen that resonates with individual health profiles, weaving together medications, lifestyle adjustments, and natural remedies into a coherent strategy that addresses symptoms while aligning with personal health philosophies. This personalization extends to the timing and dosage of treatments, where flexibility and attentiveness to one's responses guide adjustments, ensuring that the approach remains responsive to the body's changing needs.

Staying informed about new treatments is akin to charting a course through uncharted waters, where the need for caution tempers the promise of discovery. The landscape of menopause management is continually reshaped by advances in medical science, with each year bringing new treatments to the fore, from novel formulations of hormone therapy to groundbreaking non-hormonal medications that target the brain's temperature regulation centers. Engaging with this evolving field demands a proactive stance, where staying abreast of the latest studies and breakthroughs becomes a part of one's routine, like daily monitoring of symptoms or regular consultations with healthcare providers.

Discussing potential options with healthcare providers amid these advancements is a dynamic interplay of curiosity, skepticism, and hope. It requires an openness to explore emerging therapies, tempered by a critical lens that scrutinizes the evidence supporting their efficacy and safety. This dialogue is enriched by the personal data collected through symptom trackers and health diaries, offering a grounded perspective on the immediate needs and long-term goals that shape one's approach to menopause management.

Navigating the medical treatments available for menopause symptoms is a journey characterized by a meticulous examination of options, a balanced evaluation of risks and benefits, and a deep commitment to personalizing the treatment plan. It is informed by an ongoing dialogue with healthcare providers, underpinned by a proactive engagement with the latest research and innovations in the field. This approach, marked by discernment and adaptability, ensures that the strategy for managing menopause is as dynamic and individualized as the menopause experience.

6.5 The Future of Menopause Management

In the unfolding narrative of menopause management, the horizon brims with potential, signaling a future where scientific innovations and societal norms paint a new picture of this natural phase of life. Speculation about advancements in personalized medicine and innovative therapies offers a glimpse into a world where menopause care is as unique as the individuals it seeks to support. The integration of technology in tracking and managing symptoms, the momentum of advocacy for policy changes, and the evolution toward a society that openly supports menopausal women together sketch the outlines of a promising future.

The vanguard of this transformation, personalized medicine, stands poised to redefine menopause management. This approach promises treatments tailored to the individual's genetic makeup, lifestyle factors, and specific symptomatology, moving away from the one-size-fits-all paradigm. The implications are profound, with potential therapies targeting the precise hormonal imbalances or metabolic changes unique to each person. This precision enhances efficacy and minimizes side effects, making the menopausal transition smoother and more manageable. Imagine, for a moment, a scenario where a simple genetic test could guide the formulation of a hormone therapy regimen optimized for your body, mitigating risks while maximizing relief.

Parallel to the evolution of personalized medicine, technology emerges as a powerful ally in the menopause management landscape. Wearable gadgets that monitor vital signs and symptoms in real-time, apps that provide personalized wellness coaching, and online platforms that offer virtual support groups are just the beginning. These tools democratize access to health information and support, breaking down barriers of geography and removing the stigma often associated with seeking help. They also empower women to manage their symptoms actively, providing data that can inform both daily wellness choices and long-term treatment strategies.

Amidst these technological and medical advancements, a parallel movement seeks to reshape the societal and policy framework surrounding menopause. Advocacy efforts gain momentum, championing the cause for workplace accommodations such as flexible hours, temperature-controlled environments, and access to medical consultations during work hours. These changes acknowledge the impact of menopause on women's lives and validate their need for support, marking a significant shift from the silence and misunderstanding that once shrouded this phase. Furthermore, these advocacy efforts extend to healthcare access, pushing for policies that ensure comprehensive menopause care is available and affordable for all women, regardless of socioeconomic status.

Envisioning a supportive society holds the promise of open discussions about menopause, where education starts early and both men and women are informed about this natural life stage. This shift not only dispels myths and dismantles stigma but fosters an environment of empathy and support. Public health campaigns, educational programs in schools, and media portrayals that accurately reflect the menopause experience contribute to normalizing this transition, making it a topic of public conversation rather than a private struggle. In this envisioned future, menopause is not an ending but a celebrated transition, marked by wisdom, growth, and a deepened sense of self.

As we stand on the cusp of these advancements, the future of menopause management unfolds as a landscape rich with potential. From the personalized approach of medicine that promises treatments tailored to the individual through the empowering role of technology in symptom tracking and management to the societal shifts towards open support and understanding, the path forward is illuminated with hope.

Advocacy efforts that champion policy changes pave the way for a world where menopausal women receive the support and recognition they deserve, marking a leap toward a society that embraces this natural phase of life with openness and empathy.

In closing, the anticipation of what lies ahead carries with it a sense of optimism, a beacon for those navigating the menopause transition. It heralds a future where menopause management is nuanced, compassionate, and reflective of the diverse experiences of women. The convergence of medical innovation, technological support, advocacy, and societal acceptance points towards a horizon where menopause is not merely managed but embraced as a significant and empowering stage of life. As we approach the next chapter, this future vision remains a guiding light, a symbol of the progress and potential in menopause management.

7 | The Alchemy of Nutrition in Menopause

In the alchemy of managing menopause, the kitchen transforms into a laboratory, where the elements of nutrition blend to cast spells of well-being. Amidst the steam and sizzle, the ordinary act of meal preparation unfolds as a ritual, potent with the power to soothe, heal, and energize. In the crucible of our pots and pans, it's here that we discover the transformative potential of superfoods, ingredients so laden with nutrients they seem to whisper ancient secrets of health and harmony.

7.1 Superfoods for Menopause

In this culinary quest, the map to navigating menopause symptoms unfurls, revealing paths lined with salmon, berries, leafy greens, and more. Each superfood, vibrant and bursting with life, carries within it a treasure trove of vitamins, minerals, antioxidants, and omega-3 fatty acids, ready to address the body's changing needs.

Nutrient-dense Choices

In its wisdom, the body communicates its needs through the language of symptoms, craving nutrients that can recalibrate and rejuvenate. Salmon, with its rich tapestry of omega-3s, offers a balm for the inflammation that underlies many menopause symptoms, from joint stiffness to erratic moods. Berries, resplendent in their antioxidant glory, stand as guardians against oxidative stress, their vibrant hues signaling a richness that can fortify the body against cellular aging. Leafy greens, the embodiment of chlorophyll and vitamins, emerge as allies in bone health, countering the menace of osteoporosis with every crunchy, verdant bite.

The Benefits of Omega-3s

In the menopause narrative, omega-3 fatty acids emerge as heroes, wielding the dual swords of mood stabilization and inflammation reduction. The science speaks: omega-3s, particularly EPA and DHA found in fatty fish, have shown promise in mitigating the severity of hot flashes and the capriciousness of moods. As these fatty acids integrate into our meals, they weave a protective spell around our well- being, buffering us against the storms of hormonal upheaval.

Antioxidants and Menopause

The role of antioxidants in this chapter of life cannot be over-stated. Fruits and vegetables, abundant in these protective compounds, offer a shield against the oxidative stress that accelerates aging and magnifies menopause symptoms. It's a battle fought on the cellular level, where antioxidants neutralize free radicals, ensuring that each cell can function at its pinnacle, unhampered by damage or decay.

Incorporating Superfoods into Daily Meals

The alchemy of incorporating these superfoods into daily meals lies not in elaborate rituals but in simple acts of choice and preparation. Picture a morning that begins not with the haste of cereal but with the quiet assembly of a smoothie, where berries, spinach, and flaxseed oil blend into a potion of vitality. Envision transforming the humble lunch salad by crowning it with slices of grilled salmon, a drizzle of olive oil, and a scatter of walnuts, each ingredient a deliberate nod to the body's needs. Dinner becomes a canvas for creativity, where a rainbow of vegetables accompanies lean proteins, and whole grains replace yesteryear's white, refined alter- natives.

Visual Element: The Menopause Superfoods Plate

A vivid infographic, "The Menopause Superfoods Plate," illustrates how to balance a plate with these nutrient-rich foods. It divides the plate into colorful sections, each representing a category of superfoods, with annotations on the benefits of each. This visual guide serves as a daily reminder of the power of food in managing menopause symptoms, encouraging a holistic approach to meal planning that prioritizes nutrient density and variety.

In the everyday alchemy of the kitchen, where ingredients meld under the heat of our attention, food preparation transcends its routine nature, becoming a ritual of self-care and reverence for the body's journey through menopause. With each meal crafted from these superfoods, we partake in an ancient wisdom that recognizes food as medicine, a source of sustenance, healing, and balance. Through this practice, we rekindle a relationship with our bodies, learning to listen and respond with love, one meal at a time.

7.2 Understanding Phytoestrogens

In the tapestry of natural remedies for menopause, phytoestrogens emerge as subtle yet powerful threads, interwoven with the potential to ease the body's transition through hormonal shifts. These naturally occurring compounds, resembling estrogen in both form and function, weave into the fabric of plant-based foods, offering a gentle nudge towards balance in a body seeking equilibrium amidst the ebb and flow of menopause.

Phytoestrogens, in their essence, are a botanical mimicry of the body's own estrogen, engaging with estrogen receptors in a delicate ballet of hormonal interaction. These compounds in various foods, including soybeans, flaxseeds, and chick- peas, offer a natural reservoir of hormonal support. Soy, in particular, stands out for its rich isoflavone content, a class of phytoestrogens noted for their intense biological activity. With their lignans, flaxseeds offer another potent source. At the same time, chickpeas and other legumes provide a milder, though no less significant, contribution to this natural hormonal support system.

The mechanism through which phytoestrogens exert their influence is one of gentle persuasion, binding to estrogen receptors with a lighter touch than the body's own estrogen.

This interaction can serve to subtly supplement the body's dwindling estrogen levels during menopause, potentially mitigating symptoms such as hot flashes, night sweats, and the unpredictability of mood swings. It's a process that doesn't overpower or overwhelm but instead whispers to the body in a language it understands, coaxing it towards a semblance of its former hormonal harmony.

Scientific inquiry into the realm of phytoestrogens and menopause has painted a landscape rich with both promise and caution. Studies have traced the contours of phytoestrogens' potential benefits, suggesting a link between their consumption and the mitigation of menopausal symptoms. Research points to the dietary habits of populations consuming phytoestrogen-rich diets, noting a lower prevalence of menopausal discomforts, a beacon of hope for those navigating the sometimes turbulent waters of hormonal change. Yet, this research also counsels prudence, reminding us that the effects of phytoestrogens can vary widely among individuals, influenced by the complexities of each body's hormonal environment and the nuances of its metabolic pathways.

Incorporating phytoestrogens into the diet is less an act of culinary revolution and more one of thoughtful integration. It begins with the simple yet profound act of choosing whole, unprocessed foods over their refined counterparts, letting each meal become a canvas for the inclusion of phytoestrogen-rich ingredients. A sprinkle of ground flaxseeds here, a serving of soy-based yogurt there, or a hearty helping of chickpeas added to a salad; each choice is a step towards inviting phytoestrogens into the body's hormonal conversation. It's a strategy that favors moderation and variety, ensuring that these natural compounds complement rather than dominate the diet.

This approach to incorporating phytoestrogens into diets is not isolated but best nurtured within the context of a balanced and nutritious menopause-friendly diet. It acknowledges that while phytoestrogens can play a supportive role in managing menopause symptoms, they are but one piece of a more giant nutritional puzzle. When assembled with care, this puzzle supports hormonal balance. It fosters overall health, weaving together the threads of cardiovascular well- being, bone density, and emotional stability into a cohesive tapestry of menopausal health.

Ultimately, the relationship with phytoestrogens is not about seeking a panacea or a magic bullet but nurturing a dialogue with the body, listening to its needs, and responding with a diet supporting balance and well-being. It's a testament to the power of natural remedies, grounded in the earth's wisdom and the human body's resilience. It offers a path to navigate menopause with grace and vitality.

7.3 The Impact of Sugar and Processed Foods

In the intricate dance of balancing hormones during menopause, sugar, and processed foods play a role far more insidious than mere contributors to weight gain. They act as saboteurs, disrupting the delicate hormonal equilibrium and exacerbating symptoms that many strive to ease. This disruption is not an overt onslaught but a subtle undermining of the body's attempts to find balance amidst the hormonal fluctuations inherent to menopause.

Symptom Exacerbation

The consumption of high-sugar and heavily processed foods sets the stage for a cascade of physiological reactions that can amplify menopause symptoms. Hot flashes, those sudden waves of heat that wash over the body with scarcely a warning, find fertile ground in the spikes and crashes of blood sugar levels caused by sugary indulgences. Mood swings, too, akin to an unpredictable sea, are whipped into frenzied storms by the erratic energy highs and lows sugar invokes. This is not to mention the added burden on sleep quality, where sugar's interference with the body's natural sleep mechanisms can turn restorative slumber into a fitful, elusive chase.

Blood Sugar and Hormonal Balance

The link between blood sugar levels and hormonal fluctuations during menopause is a tale of intertwined destinies. Elevated blood sugar and insulin resistance, a condition where body's cells become less responsive to insulin's attempts to regulate blood sugar, can exacerbate the hormonal imbalances of menopause. Beyond its role in blood sugar regulation, insulin influences the levels of other hormones, including estrogen and progesterone. When insulin levels are persistently high, a common consequence of a diet rich in processed foods and sugars, it can contribute to the uneven hormonal terrain of menopause, making symptoms more pronounced and challenging to manage.

Healthier Alternatives

The path to mitigating these disruptions is turning towards whole, nutrient-dense foods that support rather than undermine hormonal balance. Complex carbohydrates found in whole grains, vegetables, and fruits offer a steadier source of energy, their fiber content moderating the release of glucose into the bloodstream and thus avoiding the dramatic peaks and troughs induced by their refined counterparts. Proteins and healthy fats, too, play their part, contributing to a sense of satiety, stabilizing energy levels, and providing the raw materials for hormone production and regulation. In this light, a snack of apple slices with almond butter becomes not merely a choice of preference but an act of hormonal support, a small but significant rebellion against the destabilizing influence of sugar and processed foods.

Creating a Balanced Diet Plan

Crafting a diet plan that minimizes sugar and processed foods while embracing whole, nutritious alternatives is akin to plotting a course through a labyrinth. It requires a map, a strategy, and an awareness of the traps that lie in wait. Start with the foundation—meals with vegetables, fruits, whole grains, lean proteins, and healthy fats. Each meal becomes an opportunity to nourish and support the body, with plates vibrant with the colors of a diverse range of produce, grains that provide sustained energy, and proteins and fats that contribute to hormonal and cellular health.

This does not necessitate a draconian purge of all things sweet or a banishment of convenience. Instead, it invites a shift in perspective, where sweetness is derived from natural sources, like fruits and spices, and processed foods are replaced with minimally processed alternatives that retain their nutritional integrity. Small, incremental changes and a gradual reorientation of eating habits pave the way for a sustainable transition to a menopause-friendly diet. It's a process that encourages mindfulness about food choices, fostering a connection with food beyond the superficial allure of sugar and processing to the deeper nourishment of whole foods.

In navigating this transition, the kitchen becomes a place of empowerment, a space where each ingredient is chosen for the flavor it brings to the plate and for its role in supporting the body through menopause. Recipes evolve, reflecting personal tastes and the nutritional needs of a body seeking balance. This evolution is supported by an environment that favors whole foods, where pantries and refrigerators are stocked with the tools needed to build meals that nourish and stabilize.

In this journey away from sugar and processed foods towards a diet rich in whole, nutrient-dense alternatives, the goal is not perfection but progress. It acknowledges that food is not just fuel but a key player in managing menopause symptoms. This factor can significantly ease the transition through this natural phase of life when aligned with the body's needs.

7.4 Hydration and Menopause

In the realm of bodily equilibrium during the climacteric phase, water emerges not merely as a sustainer of life but as a pivotal element in mitigating the onslaught of menopause symptoms. Its role extends beyond the simplistic act of quenching thirst, delving into the intricate processes that maintain bodily functions at their optimum. Within this context, hydration stands as a beacon, guiding the body through the tumultuous seas of hormonal fluctuations with the promise of alleviating discomforts that often accompany this life stage.

The critical nature of water in this delicate balance cannot be overstated. It serves as the medium through which nutrients travel to cells and waste products are expelled, a simple yet profound act that ensures every cellular function is performed efficiently. In the digestive labyrinth, water acts as a lubricant and a transporter, easing the passage of food through the system and thus warding off the specter of bloating and constipation that can mar the menopausal experience. Here, hydration reveals its first layer of influence, subtly yet significantly impacting the body's core operations.

Dehydration, in contrast, casts a long shadow over the menopausal landscape, exacerbating symptoms with stealth that often goes unrecognized until the effects are deeply felt. Dry skin, a common grievance as estrogen levels wane, finds little relief in the absence of adequate hydration, and the lack of moisture renders it all the more susceptible to the ravages of time and hormonal change. Vaginal dryness, too, a discomfort that whispers of the body's thirst, becomes all the more pronounced, turning intimacy into a battleground rather than a place of connection. Urinary tract infections, those unwelcome intruders, find an ally in dehydration, flourishing in conditions where a lack of fluid compromises the body's defenses to flush them out. Thus, water reveals itself as a shield, a protector against the worsening of these symptoms, offering relief in its abundance.

While seemingly straightforward, the practicalities of increasing water intake often elude strict adherence to the daily rhythm of life. Here, strategies emerge, and simple yet effective methodologies are used to ensure hydration stays within the wayside. Setting reminders, those gentle nudges in the form of alarms or apps, serve as beacons throughout the day, prompting water intake in regular intervals. This act, mechanized though it may seem, integrates the habit of hydration into the fabric of daily routines, transforming it from an act of necessity to one of subconscious compliance.

Flavoring water with fruits or herbs offers another avenue, turning the mundane act of hydration into a sensory experience. The infusion of lemon, cucumber, or mint into the water not only titillates the palate but also serves as an enticement, a beckoning towards consuming fluids that might otherwise seem unappealing in their plainness. This strategy, simple in its execution, harnesses the body's desire for variety, making the act of drinking water a pleasure rather than a chore.

Monitoring hydration levels becomes an act of attunement, a listening to the body's whispers before they crescendo into the clamor of dehydration. Signs, subtle yet telling, reveal the body's need for water. The color of urine, a spectrum that ranges from pale to dark amber, serves as a visual cue, a direct reflection of hydration levels. Dryness of the mouth, fatigue, and headaches, too, signals the body's thirst, often before conscious awareness takes hold. Adjusting fluid intake in response to these signs, increasing water consumption in response to cues, or dialing it back when hydration is adequate, requires mindfulness that attunes one to the body's rhythms and needs.

In this landscape, where hydration is pivotal in navigating the menopausal phase, its importance transcends the physical, touching on individuals' emotional and psychological well-being. The act of drinking water, deliberate and mindful, becomes a form of self-care, a recognition of the body's needs, and a commitment to meeting them. It is a practice that, while grounded in the simplicity of consuming fluids, reaches into the depths of bodily health, offering relief and support in a time of transformation.

7.5 Planning Menopause-Friendly Meals

Navigating the nutritional needs of a body in the throes of menopause demands an understanding of what to eat and an orchestrated approach to when and how these meals come together. It's an intricate dance of nutrients, timing, and portion control designed to support a body seeking balance amidst hormonal upheaval. This section unfolds the principles of assembling meals that satiate, nourish, fortify, and heal.

Meal Planning Basics

At the heart of crafting menopause-friendly meals is balancing macronutrients—proteins, fats, and carbohydrates—in a way that aligns with the body's altered metabolic rate and hormonal landscape. It's about creating a plate where each component serves a purpose, from stabilizing blood sugar levels to providing the building blocks for hormone production and mood regulation. The emphasis here shifts towards foods with a low glycemic index, lean proteins, healthy fats rich in omega-3s, and a bounty of fruits and vegetables teeming with phytonutrients and fiber. These meals become more than just food; they are a tapestry of nutrients, each thread woven to support the body's journey through menopause.

Sample Meal Ideas

Breakfast might see the dawn of a new day with a bowl of steel-cut oats, simmered gently and served with a sprinkle of chia seeds, walnuts, and a generous handful of blueberries. This meal, rich in fiber, omega-3s, and antioxidants, kickstarts the day on a note of balanced blood sugar and sustained energy. For lunch, envision a salad that's a kaleidoscope of colors: dark leafy greens, vibrant bell peppers, avocado slices, and quinoa, dressed lightly with olive oil and lemon juice. Such a meal not only delights the palate but floods the body with vitamins, minerals, and healthy fats, crucial for cellular health and hormonal balance.

Dinner could unfold as a symphony of flavors, with grilled salmon taking center stage, accompanied by a medley of roasted vegetables and a side of farro. This combination, rich in protein, omega-3 fatty acids, and complex carbohydrates, satisfies the taste buds and supports heart health, bone density, and emotional well-being. Snacks, often overlooked, play a vital role in maintaining energy levels and preventing blood sugar dips. A handful of almonds or a slice of apple with almond butter offers a quick, nutritious boost, keeping hunger and mood swings at bay.

Adjusting Portion Sizes

With the metabolic shifts that accompany menopause, the adage "less is more" finds new relevance. Portion control becomes a critical tool in managing weight and symptoms. This practice entails listening to the body's cues of hunger and fullness rather than adhering to preset portion sizes. This mindfulness allows for an adjustment in food intake that reflects the body's actual needs, which may fluctuate daily. It's a gentle approach that respects the body's wisdom and fosters a harmonious relationship with food.

Involving Family in Meal Planning

Creating menopause-friendly meals should be a collaborative endeavor, and it should alienate those we share our tables with. Involving family members in meal planning and preparation can transform this journey into a shared adventure where nutritional goals align with the pleasure of eating together. It's an opportunity to educate, explore new foods and flavors, and cultivate a family-wide appreciation for meals supporting well-being at every life stage. This inclusivity not only eases the mealtime dynamics but also rein- forces the support system, a network of understanding and care that is crucial during menopause.

As this chapter on meal planning draws to a close, it leaves us with a vision of food as more than mere sustenance. In the context of menopause, every meal becomes an opportunity to nourish the body, ease symptoms, and embrace the changes with strength and resilience. Through thoughtful planning, a focus on nutrient-rich foods, and the mindful adjustment of portion sizes, we find not just health but a deeper connection to the rhythms of our bodies. And as we share these meals with those we love, we weave a more substantial fabric of support, understanding, and care, setting the stage for the chapters yet to unfold.

8 | Reframing Movement for Menopause

In the landscape of menopause, where hormonal shifts sculpt new terrains within the body, the act of moving—intentional, mindful movement—becomes a potent tool for sculpting back, a way to mold resilience from within. It's not about high stakes, all-or-nothing gambles on physical prowess but rather a gentle recalibration of how and why we move. This nuanced approach to exercise during menopause doesn't just address the symptoms; it rewires the body's response to them, layering benefits that extend beyond the immediate relief into the realm of long-term well-being.

8.1 The Best Exercises for Menopause

The Types of Beneficial Exercises

The spectrum of beneficial exercises during menopause is broad, inviting a tailored approach that respects the body's current narrative. Cardiovascular activities, those rhythmic, repetitive movements that mount the heart rate, stand tall for their dual role in symptom management and cardiovascular health. Walking, cycling, and swimming emerge as champions, accessible yet powerful; they weave endurance into the fabric of daily life, reducing the frequency of hot flashes, improving sleep, and uplifting mood.

Often overlooked in the feminine fitness lexicon, strength training demands its due recognition. Lifting weights, whether dumbbells, resistance bands, or the body's own weight, builds muscle and fortitude against osteoporosis, a shadow that looms post-menopause. The empowerment found in growing more robust, in watching one's own capacity expand, is a testament to the body's adaptability and its potential for renewal.

Flexibility exercises, including stretching, targeted movement practices, and a whisper of balance and grace, are vital in a phase where the body seeks harmony. They lengthen and loosen, easing the stiffness that creeps into joints and muscles, promoting a fluidity of movement that mirrors a fluidity of spirit.

Customizing Exercise Routines

Customization is critical, turning exercise from a prescribed routine into a personal rhythm that resonates with the individual's life. It's about finding what fits, what sparks joy, and what sustains motivation. For some, it might be a morning walk, where each step is a meditation, an attunement to the day. For others, it could be a dance class where the music and movement dissolve the world's weight or a cycling class where the challenge is not just the terrain but the boundaries of one's own stamina.

Benefits Beyond Symptom Relief

The tapestry of benefits woven by regular exercise in menopause's context extends into the rich landscape of bone density, heart health, and mental well-being. Each movement, each effort, deposits into the bank of long-term health, building reserves that guard against the risk of heart disease, diabetes, and cognitive decline. It's an investment in the future, in a vision of aging that defies the stereotype of fragility, championing vitality instead.

Starting Points for Beginners

For those at the threshold, the beginners, starting points are beacons of light. It's about setting the bar where it's reachable, celebrating small victories, and gradually stretching the limits. Initiating this journey with a walk, the simplicity of putting one foot in front of the other, offers a gateway to larger realms of movement. The key is consistency, finding a rhythm that can be sustained, and then, layer by layer, adding complexity and challenge.

Visual Element: Exercise Selection Wheel

The Exercise Selection Wheel, a visual element, offers a colorful guide to choosing activities tailored to menopause's diverse needs. It has three parts: cardiovascular, strength, and flexibility exercises. This wheel spins a narrative of choice, encouraging women to mix and match activities that resonate with their preferences and goals. Each segment details exercises within its domain, providing a tactile, engaging tool for crafting a personalized exercise blueprint.

In menopause's landscape, the reframing movement becomes a narrative of empowerment, a way to reclaim agency over a body in flux. It's about moving with intention, crafting routines that not just alleviate symptoms but enrich the entirety of one's being. Through customized routines, mindful choices, and an eye on the holistic benefits, exercise trans- forms into a dialogue with the body that nurtures and sustains.

8.2 Yoga and Pilates for Hormonal Health

In the tapestry of strategies woven to mitigate the multifaceted symptoms of menopause, both yoga and Pilates emerge as threads of gold, their effectiveness undimmed by the passage of time. These practices, rooted in balance and centering principles, invite a dialogue with the body that transcends mere physicality, touching on the essence of seeking equilibrium in times of change. These disciplines' gentle yet profound nature offers a refuge from the storm and a means to navigate it with a sense of serenity and strength.

Cultivating a mind-body connection through yoga and Pilates is more than a symbolic bridge linking thought to action or intention to movement. It is a concrete pathway through which awareness becomes as fluid as the movements them- selves, facilitating a deeper understanding of the body's signals and needs. In the realm of menopause, where the body seems at times to speak a foreign tongue, this connection becomes invaluable. Through the focused breathwork of yoga or Pilates' precise, controlled movements, individuals find a means to ground themselves, to listen intently to what lies beneath the surface of transient symptoms. This attentive- ness fosters a reduction in stress and a profound sense of balance that tempers emotional fluctuations and brings clarity to a mind besieged by the fog of hormonal upheaval.

Specific poses and exercises within these disciplines hold keys to unlocking relief from menopause's grip. In yoga, the cooling breath (Sitali Pranayama) acts as a balm for the heat of hot flashes, while poses like the Supported Bridge or Seated Forward Bend gently coax the body into a state of relaxation, easing tension and countering insomnia. Pilates, emphasizing core strength, offers physical and metaphorical stability, fortifying the body against shifting hormones. The pelvic floor engagement in Pilates, a focus that mirrors yoga's attention to the body's energetic centers, supports urinary health, an aspect of menopause often cloaked in silence but keenly felt by many.

Incorporating mindfulness into the practice of yoga and Pilates serves as a lantern lighting the way through menopause's darker moments. Mindfulness, the art of being wholly present, transforms each stretch and pose into a meditation in motion. It teaches the practitioner to fully inhabit their body and experience each sensation without judgment or anticipation. This presence of mind extends beyond the mat, influencing reactions to stress and emotional disturbances off it. Through mindfulness, the tumultuous waves of menopause are met with a stability that is as much about emotional resilience as it is about physical balance. The practice becomes a sanctuary, a space where the storms of the outside world are met with calmness and where hormonal upheavals are greeted with grace.

For those beginning their journey with yoga and Pilates, the landscape is rich with resources designed to ease the initiation. Beginner-friendly classes, whether found in the local studio or through online platforms, offer an accessible entry point, guiding novices through the foundational poses and principles with patience and care. These classes, often marked by a focus on gentle or restorative practices, cater to the unique needs of the menopausal body, acknowledging its limitations and celebrating its capabilities. Online resources abound, from instructional videos that break down each pose with clarity and compassion to digital communities that offer support and encouragement. These resources, whether tapped into from the privacy of one's living room or as part of a group class, demystify the practices of yoga and Pilates, making them approachable and relatable.

In this rich field of movement and mindfulness, yoga and Pilates stand as beacons for those navigating the hormonal shifts of menopause. They offer a strategy for managing symptoms and practice deep listening and response to harmonize the body's rhythms with the natural cycles of change. Through these disciplines, individuals find relief and a profound sense of connection to themselves, providing grounding during this significant transition.

8.3 The Importance of Consistency and Moderation

In the tapestry of menopause management, the threads of consistency and moderation weave through the fabric of exercise routines, not as mere embellishments but as foundational elements vital for creating a harmonious whole. Culturing these principles within the context of physical activity is akin to tending a garden with care and precision, ensuring each plant thrives without overshadowing its neighbors, each receiving just the right amount of sunlight and water to flourish. In this delicate balance, the garden of well-being blooms, sustained by the rhythms of regularity and the wisdom of restraint.

Setting Achievable Fitness Goals

In a physical activity, setting goals serves as the compass by which direction is determined, guiding the traveler through familiar and uncharted landscapes. Yet, the art of goal-setting transcends the mere selection of destinations; it requires an intimate understanding of one's capacities and limitations, an acknowledgment of the current state of the body's landscape, marked by the ebbs and flows of menopausal symptoms. Achievable goals acknowledge this reality and recognize the virtue in small, incremental steps forward. They are beacons that light the path, not with the blinding glare of ambition, but with the soft glow of attainability. In this light, the traveler moves forward, each step a testament to progress, each milestone a celebration of capability.

The Role of Rest and Recovery

Within the exercise cycle, rest emerges not as a passive state but as an active participant in the journey toward well-being. It is the soil where recovery takes root, the space in which muscles mend and the spirit rejuvenates. The inclusion of rest days in exercise routines acknowledges the body's need for this respite, for moments of stillness in which the work of healing can occur. It is an understanding that strength lies not just in action but in the quiet that follows, that the body's whispers of fatigue are not to be ignored but honored. This respect for rest and recovery prevents the encroachment of injury and the fatigue that can derail the best-laid plans, ensuring the sustainability of the exercise journey.

Listening to Your Body

The dialogue between body and mind becomes particularly poignant in menopause, a period characterized by the body's fluent expression of its needs and discomforts. Tuning into this communication requires a keen awareness and a willingness to hear what is often unspoken. It involves deciphering the body's language of symptoms and recognizing when to push forward and when to pull back. Adjusting exercise intensity and duration in response to the body's signals is not a sign of retreat but of intelligent navigation. This skill ensures the journey continues and does so in a manner that respects the body's changing landscapes. This attunement to the body's needs fosters a relationship of trust and cooperation, where physical activity becomes a dialogue, a give-and- take that sustains and nurtures.

Building a Sustainable Routine

Constructing a sustainable exercise routine is an act of architecture that requires both vision and pragmatism. It asks for a blueprint that considers the foundation—current levels of fitness and the impact of menopausal symptoms—while also allowing for the flexibility to adapt and evolve. Building this routine is less about erecting a tower in haste and more about laying each brick with intention, considering how today's choices will stand the test of time. It involves integrating exercise into the fabric of daily life, making it as intrinsic to the day as meals and sleep. This integration ensures that physical activity is not an interloper, demanding time and space with the weight of obligation, but a welcome and familiar presence, woven into the patterns of the day with ease and grace. Tips for this construction include:

- ↻ Selecting activities that bring joy.
- ↻ Scheduling exercises as one would a necessary appointment.
- ↻ Celebrating the consistency of effort over the fluctuation of intensity.

In this way, the routine becomes sustainable, a structure built to endure the challenges of menopause and beyond, offering shelter and strength in equal measure.

In navigating the menopausal transition, the principles of consistency and moderation in exercise offer a counterpoint to the turbulence of symptoms, a steadying force in change. They advocate an approach that values gradual progress over immediate results, understands the restorative power of rest, and listens attentively to the body's evolving needs. This approach, grounded in the rhythms of regularity and the wisdom of restraint, ensures that the journey through menopause is not just endured but embraced, with each step forward marked by a sense of achievement and well-being.

8.4 Overcoming Barriers to Exercise

Recognizing and dismantling personal barriers is pivotal in maintaining physical activity during menopause. Reflection unveils these hurdles, often masquerading as mere inconveniences—time constraints echo the relentless pace of daily obligations, a dwindling spark of motivation whispers of deeper emotional battles, and physical limitations cast shadows of doubt on capabilities. Acknowledgment is the first stride towards empowerment, a silent nod to the self that these barriers, though formidable, are not insurmountable.

Strategies to rekindle the flame of motivation are manifold, each a beacon guiding through the fog of reluctance. The art of setting small, digestible goals transforms the mountain of aspiration into a series of manageable hills, each ascent a victory in its own right. This segmentation of the journey into quantifiable achievements fuels a sense of progression, a tangible measure of advancement that, bit by bit, constructs a narrative of triumph. In parallel, the cultivation of social support serves as both a mirror and a catalyst, reflecting back the potential for success and propelling forward with the momentum of collective energy. Whether found in the flesh or within the digital ether of online communities, exercise partners morph into allies, their presence a constant reminder of shared aspirations and mutual encouragement. Diversifying activities introduce a palette of possibilities, turning routine into exploration. Switching between different forms of exercise keeps the body guessing. The mind is engaged, and each new activity is a chapter in a broader story of physical discovery.

Adapting exercises to accommodate the unique tapestry of menopause symptoms requires a nuanced understanding of the body's language. It's an intimate conversation that listens for the whispers of discomfort and responds with modifications that respect the body's current dialogue. High-impact routines evolve into their low-impact counterparts, their essence preserved. Still, their form transformed to reduce strain on joints and alleviate the pressure of exertion. Flexibility and strength training merge, their union offering a foundation that supports the body's core while gently stretching its limits. This tailored approach does not concede to symptoms. Instead, it negotiates with them, finding a middle ground where exercise remains a source of strength and rejuvenation.

Integrating technology into the scaffolding of exercise routines offers a bridge across the chasm of isolation. Fitness apps become personal trainers, residing in the pocket or on the wrist, their reminders and trackers a constant companion on the journey. These digital tools offer a blend of account- ability and personalization, precisely tracking progress and tailoring recommendations to the user's evolving needs. Online communities serve as virtual gyms, spaces where encouragement and advice flow freely, untethered by the constraints of geography. Virtual classes break down the barriers of time and location, bringing the guidance of instructors into the living room, their expertise a click away. This melding of technology and fitness crafts a web of support that is accessible and responsive, ensuring that the path of physical activity, though walked alone, is far from lonely.

In this intricate web of strategies, barriers to exercise, from insurmountable walls to daunting hurdles, can be overcome with patience and creativity. The journey through menopause, marked by its physical and emotional fluctuations, demands not just the acknowledgment of these barriers but a commitment to their dismantling. By setting achievable goals, fostering social support, embracing diverse activities, and leveraging technology, exercise reclaims its place not as a chore but as a cherished ally in the quest for balance and well-being. This approach, rooted in adaptation and resilience, ensures that physical activity remains a steadfast companion through the menopausal transition, a source of strength, vitality, and renewal.

8.5 Measuring the Impact of Exercise on Symptoms

In the nuanced dance of aligning physical exertion with the ebbs and flows of menopausal symptoms, meticulous tracking emerges as an invaluable ally. This practice, akin to charting the stars to navigate vast oceans, involves a dual focus: diligently recording each amount of physical activity alongside the fluctuating landscape of menopause symptoms. Such diligent documentation illuminates patterns previously shrouded in the complexity of bodily responses, revealing the intricate interplay between movement and well-being. For those navigating the unpredictable waters of menopause, this approach offers a beacon of clarity, guiding adjustments to exercise regimens with precision and insight.

Tracking Symptoms and Activities

Embarking on this analytical journey necessitates tools that capture the full spectrum of experiences, from the intensity and duration of physical activities to the subtleties of symptom fluctuations. Digital apps, with their capacity for detailed logs and real-time tracking, stand out for their convenience and comprehensiveness, serving as modern-day compasses in this exploratory process. Yet, the tactile nature of pen and paper holds its charm, offering a canvas for reflections that transcend mere data, capturing the emotional hues of each day. Regardless of the medium, the act of tracking becomes a ritual, a daily engagement with the self that fosters a deeper understanding of the body's narratives. Though grounded in the mundane, this practice transcends its logistical nature, transforming routine logs into a rich tapestry of insights that guide the journey through menopause with informed intention.

Adjusting Based on Feedback

Armed with the insights gleaned from meticulous tracking, the path forward beckons, illuminated by the light of personal data. Here, the art of adjustment takes center stage, demanding informed and intuitive responsiveness. It is not about adhering rigidly to prescribed routines but about dancing with the data, allowing it to lead as symptoms and responses unfold. Perhaps the revelation that certain activities exacerbate hot flashes prompts a shift towards cooler, less intense workouts. Or the discovery that yoga imbues body flexibility and mood stability and encourages its integration into daily routines. This responsive approach, rooted in the feedback loop of tracking and adjusting, ensures that exercise serves not as a static prescription but as a dynamic, evolving component of menopause management.

Celebrating Progress

Within this framework of observation and adaptation, progress unfurls, often in subtle increments that might elude notice without the keen eye of documentation. Celebrating these advancements, whether they manifest as a reduction in symptom severity, an increase in energy levels, or a newfound joy in movement, becomes vital. It's a practice acknowledging the effort invested, the resilience displayed, and the victories achieved, regardless of scale. Recognizing progress serves not just as a reward but as a reinforcement, a reminder of the power inherent in consistent, mindful engagement with exercise. This acknowledgment, whether shared with supportive communities or savored in solitary reflection, weaves a thread of positivity through the menopause narrative, spotlighting the capacity for growth and adaptation even amidst challenges.

Sharing Success Stories

In the shared space of communal journeys, success stories resonate with a unique power, echoing the triumphs of individual paths while lighting the way for others. Inviting those navigating menopause to share their tales of triumph in integrating exercise into their lives serves multiple purposes. It democratizes knowledge, transforming personal insights into communal wisdom. It fosters a spirit of solidarity, reminding each collective member that they are not alone in their struggles or successes. Moreover, it catalyzes motivation, illustrating through lived experiences the tangible benefits of aligning movement with menopausal well-being. These narratives, rich in diversity and depth, contribute to a mosaic of menopause management strategies, each story a testament to the transformative potential of exercise.

In menopause management, exercise integration emerges as a beacon of agency amidst the fluctuating terrain of symptoms. In menopause management, exercise integration emerges as a beacon of agency amidst the fluctuating terrain of symptoms. Through the meticulous tracking of physical activities and the corresponding ebb and flow of symptoms, individuals carve paths of personalized adjustment guided by the unique narratives of their bodies. Celebrating progress, in all its forms, reinforces the journey, imbuing it with a sense of achievement and possibility. Sharing these tales of triumph weaves a tapestry of communal wisdom, highlighting the collective power of individual journeys. This chapter, though singular in its focus, is interwoven with the overarching narrative of navigating menopause with informed grace, each stride forward illuminated by the insights gleaned from a dialogue between movement and well-being. As we turn the page, the journey continues, each step a testament to the resilience and adaptability that define the menopausal transition.

In this realm beyond symptoms, the survivors underscore the significance of nurturing the body and spirit with continued attention to nutrition and physical activity, tailored now not to the management of menopause but to the celebration of vitality. They advocate maintaining the social connections forged in the crucible of transition, for these bonds, tempered by shared experience, hold a depth and resilience that enrich life in profound ways.

The tapestry of advice and insight these long-term survivors share weaves a narrative of hope and resilience. It offers a roadmap through the shifting terrain of menopause, marked by practical strategies for managing symptoms and enriched by a perspective that sees beyond the immediate to the promise of what lies ahead. Their wisdom, born of experience, stands as a testament to the capacity for adaptation, growth, and renewal that defines not just the menopause transition but the journey of life itself.

9 Cultivating Calm in the Menopause Maelstrom

In the orchestra of life's transitions, menopause holds its own unique melody, a composition that, while inherently beautiful, carries complexities that demand both attention and intention. Within this symphony, mindfulness and meditation emerge not as mere background music but as powerful instruments, capable of transforming dissonance into harmony. The practice of tuning into the present, of finding stillness amidst the whirlwind of hormonal change, offers a profound counterpoint to the often turbulent experience of menopause.

9.1 Mindfulness and Meditation for Menopause

Introduction to Mindfulness and Meditation

According to Jon Kabat-Zinn, Mindfulness, the act of nonjudgmentally paying attention to purpose in the present moment, forms the cornerstone of a practice that roots us in the 'now.' Its counterpart, meditation, offers a structured approach to cultivating this awareness through techniques ranging from focused breathing to guided imagery. Together, they form a duo that speaks directly to the heart of menopause management, addressing not just the physical symptoms but the emotional landscape accompanying this life stage.

Techniques for Beginners

For those new to this practice, the beginning might be setting aside five minutes each morning, sitting in a quiet space, and simply observing the breath. Inhale, exhale, notice the rise and fall of the chest, the sensation of air moving through the nostrils. When thoughts intrude, as they inevitably will, the practice isn't to banish them but to acknowledge their presence and gently guide attention back to the breath. This simple daily act serves as a foundational exercise in mindful- ness, a stepping stone towards more profound meditation practices.

Imagine integrating mindfulness into everyday activities, transforming mundane tasks into moments of meditation. During a walk, for instance, attention might shift to the sensation of footfalls on the earth, the rhythm of breathing, or the symphony of sounds that fill the air. Here, mindfulness weaves itself into the fabric of daily life, offering pockets of calm and presence.

Benefits for Menopause Symptoms

The regular practice of mindfulness and meditation offers a buffer against the stress that often exacerbates menopause symptoms. Studies have shown that stress can heighten the intensity of hot flashes and disrupt sleep patterns, making stress management through mindfulness an attractive strategy for symptom relief. Additionally, the cultivation of a mindful approach to life can temper mood swings and foster a sense of emotional equilibrium, offering a steadying influence amidst the hormonal flux of menopause.

Resources for Deeper Exploration

For those eager to explore further, a wealth of resources awaits. Apps like Headspace and Calm provide guided meditations tailored to various needs and experiences, including stress reduction, sleep improvement, and emotional balance. Books such as *The Miracle of Mindfulness* by Thich Nhat Hanh offer insights into mindfulness practice. At the same time, online courses provide structured paths to deepening one's meditation practice.

Visual Element: The Mindfulness Meditation Wheel

A visual guide, "The Mindfulness Meditation Wheel," is a compass for beginners, delineating various techniques and practices that anchor mindfulness in daily life. This wheel is segmented into areas such as Breath Focus, Body Scan, Mindful Movement, and Loving-Kindness Meditation, each section offering a brief description and tips for integration. Accompanying the wheel, a set of guided prompts encourages reflection on the experience of each practice, fostering an interactive exploration of mindfulness and meditation.

In the shifting landscape of menopause, mindfulness, and meditation stand as beacons of calm, tools that, when wielded with intention, can illuminate the path through this transformative phase. They invite a dialogue with the present, encouraging a deep listening to the body's wisdom and the heart's whispers. Through this practice, the experience of menopause can be not just navigated but embraced, its challenges met with stability, and its gifts received with gratitude.

9.2 Cognitive Behavioral Therapy (CBT) and Menopause

Explaining CBT

Cognitive Behavioral Therapy (CBT) emerges within the therapeutic landscape as a beacon of clarity, asserting that the triad of thoughts, feelings, and behaviors is interconnected and dynamically interactive. It posits that our cognitive processes— how we interpret and understand our world— profoundly influence our emotional state and subsequent actions. Within this framework, CBT doesn't just spotlight the symptom, it also delves into the narrative behind it, peeling back the layers to reveal cognitive distortions that may amplify distress or discomfort. By adjusting these perceptions and interpretations, CBT aims to recalibrate emotional responses and foster more adaptive behaviors, introducing a level of agency that might have felt elusive to those caught in the cyclical storm of menopause symptoms.

CBT for Menopause Symptom Management

In the specific application of CBT to menopause, this therapy adapts its focus, homing in on the symptoms that often accompany this period of transition—particularly anxiety, depression, and sleep disturbances. This is not a matter of mere symptom chasing but an acknowledgment of the intricate web in which physical changes and psychological states entangle during menopause. For instance, hot flashes may not just be a physical sensation but carry a psychological weight, burdened with anxiety about their occurrence and impact. CBT steps in as a mediator, offering strategies to reframe these experiences, reducing the anticipatory anxiety that often exacerbates the symptom itself. Through structured sessions, women learn to identify and challenge the catastrophizing thoughts that might accompany a hot flash or the pervasive belief that sleep will inevitably be elusive, replacing these with more balanced, evidence-based perspectives. This process, iterative and reflective, works to diminish the intensity of menopause's emotional and psychological toll, fostering a sense of resilience and empowerment.

Finding a CBT Therapist

Securing the guidance of a skilled CBT therapist, one versed in the nuances of menopause, is akin to finding a navigator for uncharted waters. It demands diligence and compatibility, ensuring that this therapeutic alliance is both knowledgeable and empathetic. Initiating this search might involve consultations with healthcare providers for referrals or engaging with professional psychology directories that filter practitioners by specialization and location. While it may require patience, the selection process is pivotal, underpinned by the under- standing that the therapeutic relationship itself is a corner- stone of effective treatment. Dialogues with potential therapists should illuminate their familiarity with menopause as a focus area, their approach to therapy, and their perspective on the interplay between physical and psychological symptoms.

Self-help CBT Strategies

For those who find themselves navigating this landscape independently, either by choice or necessity, CBT offers a trove of self-help strategies that can be harnessed with autonomy. Central to this is the practice of self-monitoring—keeping a detailed diary that tracks not only menopause symptoms but the thoughts and emotions that accompany them. This diary becomes a mirror, reflecting patterns and triggers that might otherwise remain obscured. Equipped with this insight, individuals can begin the work of cognitive restructuring on their own, identifying negative or distorted thought patterns and challenging them with evidence and balanced thinking. Techniques such as 'behavioral activation,' which encourages engagement with activities that boost mood and counteract withdrawal, can be self-initiated, fostering a sense of engagement with life that menopause might have dimmed.

Digital and print resources abound for those seeking to apply CBT principles independently. Workbooks grounded in CBT offer structured exercises that guide users through the process of identifying cognitive distortions, practicing alternative thought generation, and gradually confronting feared situations in a controlled, step-by-step manner. Online platforms and mobile applications designed around CBT principles provide interactive tools for mood tracking, cognitive restructuring exercises, and stress management techniques, all tailored to the user's specific needs and symptoms.

In threading CBT into the fabric of menopause management, a dual pathway emerges that acknowledges and addresses the physiological realities of this transition while untangling the psychological responses that amplify its challenges. This approach does not negate the physicality of menopause. Still, it adds a layer of cognitive and emotional resilience, offering a strategy that is as much about redefining the experience of menopause as it is about managing its symptoms. Through the deliberate application of CBT, either within the therapeutic setting or through self- guided efforts, individuals find a means to navigate menopause not as a period of loss but as an opportunity for growth, adaptation, and empowerment.

9.3 The Power of Positive Thinking

In the intricate dance of navigating menopause, the power of positive thinking emerges as a beacon, illuminating paths through the oft-shadowed realms of this transition. This isn't merely about wearing rose-colored glasses; it is about engaging in a deliberate practice that reshapes the narrative of menopause from one of loss to a period ripe with potential. In this context, positive thinking becomes a tool that meticulously carves out spaces of light in the denser forests of change, reminding us that how we perceive our experiences significantly colors their impact on our lives.

The influence of adopting a positive outlook extends its roots deep into the soil of mental and emotional health, offering nourishment that fosters resilience against the sometimes harsh winds of menopause. Here, focusing on the growth potential, the opportunity for introspection, and the possibility of renewal counterbalances to the weight of hot flashes, mood swings, and the myriad other symptoms accompanying this transition. It's a practice that acknowledges the challenges but refuses to be defined by them, instead highlighting the strength, wisdom, and grace accompanying this phase of life.

Cultivating positivity, however, demands more than a fleeting wish or a passive hope; it requires active engagement through techniques designed to tilt the scales from negativity to a more balanced, affirmative perspective. Gratitude journaling stands out as a cornerstone practice, a daily ritual where one lists, without fail, aspects of their life for which they are thankful. This could range from the seemingly mundane—a warm cup of tea, a moment of silence before the day begins— to the profound, such as the support of friends or the beauty of experiencing another day. This practice trains the mind to seek out and acknowledge the positive, gradually shifting the default setting from one of deficit to one of abundance.

Positive affirmations, coupled with gratitude, offer another layer of reinforcement. These short, powerful statements, framed in the present tense and spoken with conviction, remind one of one's worth, strength, and capability. "I am navigating menopause with strength and patience," for instance, becomes not just a sentence but a mantra, a declaration that shapes reality through repetition and belief. Over time, these affirmations seep into the subconscious, subtly altering self-perception and the perception of menopause itself.

Yet, the path to positive thinking is sometimes strewn with the debris of negative self-talk, those inner dialogues that critique and diminish, often without our conscious consent. Identifying these patterns is the first step in dismantling them, which demands vigilance and honesty. Once recognized, the strategy shifts to challenging these narratives, questioning their validity, and reframing them in a more positive or realistic light. This doesn't mean denying difficulties but instead refusing to let them define the entirety of the menopause experience. It's a method of disempowering the negativity that can cloud this transition, clearing the skies for a more nuanced understanding of menopause, one that includes but is not limited to its challenges.

Surrounding oneself with positive influences and support amplifies the impact of individual practices, creating an environment where positive thinking can flourish. Whether composed of friends, family, support groups, or online communities, this network acts as a mirror, reflecting the potential for a positive menopause experience. Conversations within these circles that highlight triumphs, share strategies for coping, and offer encouragement act as lifelines, pulling focus away from the solitary struggle and towards a collective journey marked by understanding and mutual support.

In engaging with these practices—gratitude journaling, positive affirmations, challenging negative self-talk, and building a supportive network—the landscape of menopause transforms. No longer a monolith of loss and discomfort, it becomes a mosaic, rich with complexity and beauty, where challenges exist but do not dominate. In this light, positive thinking isn't an act of naivety but a radical act of rebalance. It is a way to hold space for the menopause experience without being overwhelmed by its more challenging aspects.

9.4 Emotional Resilience Building

Understanding Emotional Resilience

In menopause's fluctuating landscape, emotional resilience is a beacon of internal strength. This quality allows one to weather the storms of change with a certain poise. This resilience, far from being an innate trait bestowed upon the lucky few, emerges as a skill cultivated over time, through conscious effort and deliberate practice. It embodies the capacity to bounce back from the emotional ebbs. It flows characteristic of menopause and stands amidst the uncertainty with a steadfast heart. The significance of this resilience cannot be overstated; it transforms how one navigates the challenges, turning potential stumbling blocks into stepping stones, each an opportunity for growth and deeper self-understanding.

Emotional resilience during menopause means recognizing that while the physical symptoms may ebb and flow, control over one's emotional response remains firmly within grasp. It is about cultivating a space of inner calm that can be returned to time and again despite the external chaos. This inner sanctuary becomes a source of strength, a wellspring of tranquility that supports one through the unpredictable waves of hormonal change.

Strategies for Building Resilience

The architecture of emotional resilience is both intricate and personal, yet specific universal strategies serve as its pillars. The pursuit of social support emerges as a critical component, a reminder that though the menopause experience is deeply personal, it need not be solitary. Engaging with friends, family, or support groups who provide empathy, understanding, and shared experience can lighten the emotional load, making the burdens less demanding to bear alone. These connections remind us that our struggles are shared and that there is strength in vulnerability and immense power in collective empathy.

Practicing self-care evolves as another fundamental strategy, a tangible manifestation of self-compassion that acknowledges the body and mind's need for rest, nourishment, and nurturing. Self-care during menopause might translate into prioritizing sleep, indulging in activities that bring joy and relaxation, or simply allowing oneself moments of stillness amidst the daily hustle. It is a conscious act of turning inward, and of listening and responding to the body's needs with kindness and care—a direct counteraction to the stressors that threaten emotional equilibrium.

Setting healthy boundaries is equally crucial, a practice that involves discerning and asserting one's limits in both personal and professional spheres. It means saying no without guilt, seeking balance to prevent burnout, and protecting one's energy with the same vigilance as one's physical health. In the context of menopause, where emotional reserves may fluctuate, these boundaries become lifelines, preserving a sense of self amidst the myriad demands of daily life.

Learning from Challenges

Viewing menopause-related challenges as occasions for growth and learning enhances personal resilience. This perspective shift reframes obstacles as teachers, each symptom or difficulty a lesson in understanding, adapting, and ultimately thriving. It encourages a stance of curiosity rather than resistance, an openness to exploring what each experience offers regarding insight into oneself and one's capacity for adaptation. This learning stance fosters resilience by transforming the narrative around menopause from struggle to empowerment and growth.

Resources for Resilience Training

For those seeking to deepen their well of emotional resilience, a plethora of resources awaits. Books that delve into the science and art of resilience, such as "The Resilience Factor" by Karen Reivich and Andrew Shatté, offer strategies grounded in psychological research, providing readers with tools to build and maintain resilience. Workshops and seminars dedicated to resilience training present opportunities for experiential learning, often incorporating practices from mindfulness, CBT, and positive psychology into their curricula. These settings equip participants with resilience-building techniques and foster a sense of community among attendees, reinforcing the importance of social support in resilience cultivation.

Online platforms and digital applications focusing on mental well-being and emotional resilience provide accessible avenues for exploration and practice. These resources often feature interactive elements, such as guided meditations, journaling prompts, and personalized activities designed to strengthen emotional resilience. Engaging with these digital tools allows for a customized approach to resilience training, enabling users to integrate practices into their daily routines at their own pace.

In exploring emotional resilience during menopause, a multifaceted approach emerges that intertwines social support, self-care, boundary setting, and a learning stance. Each strategy, resource, and practice contribute to the construction of a robust emotional foundation, one capable of withstanding the fluctuations of menopause with grace and strength; by actively cultivating this resilience, the experience of menopause shifts, marked not by the challenges it presents but by the growth, understanding, and empowerment it fosters.

9.5 Managing Anxiety and Depression

In the tapestry of menopause, threads of anxiety and depression often weave through, subtly altering the pattern with their presence. Amidst the flux of hormonal shifts, recognizing the signs of these unwelcome guests becomes a subtle art. Symptoms may dress themselves in the cloak of menopause's myriad changes. Yet, they carry a distinct weight, casting longer shadows that linger beyond the momentary. Palpitations, a relentless sense of dread, an exhaustion that sleep does not ease, and a joylessness that colors days grey—these markers serve as signposts, signaling a terrain that demands navigation with care.

The path to managing these symptoms begins with lifestyle modifications, not as panaceas but as significant allies in the broader strategy. Once a mere footnote in the day's agenda, physical activity rises as a stalwart defender, its rhythmic consistency countering anxiety's erratic pulse. The alchemy of exercise releases a cascade of endorphins, nature's salve, soothing frayed nerves and lifting spirits with its natural buoyancy. Nutrition, too, asserts its role in this equilibrium. Meals become mindful choices, plates balanced not just in calories but in nutrients that fortify the mind as much as the body—omega-3-rich foods, leafy greens, and whole grains are foundations, supporting neural pathways and emotional stability. Sleep hygiene, often disrupted in the menopause maelstrom, demands a recommitment to rituals that invite rest—dimmed lights, cooled rooms, and the gentle disengagement from screens and stresses that prelude slumber.

Yet, there are times when the weight of anxiety and depression refuses to lift, rooted deeply in the psyche, unswayed by the well-intentioned efforts of lifestyle adjustments. In these moments, seeking professional help becomes not a sign of defeat but an act of profound self-care. Therapists and counselors, skilled in navigating the nuances of mental health, offer not just interventions but understanding, a space where the complexities of menopause, mental health, and individual experience are acknowledged and addressed. This professional guidance, tailored to the individual, illuminates paths forward, through the dense underbrush of anxiety and depression, towards more evident ground.

Supportive therapies and treatments unfold as a spectrum of options, each with its own merits. Counseling, a dialogue rooted in empathy, provides a reflective surface, a means to see one's experience through the lens of objectivity and compassion. Medication, when recommended, acts as a bridge, carrying one over tumultuous waters to more stable ground—it is a tool, used with discretion, that can recalibrate the chemical imbalances that often underpin depression and anxiety. Alternative therapies introduce a holistic dimension, such as acupuncture, aromatherapy, and herbal supplements weaving through the care regimen with complementary colors, adding depth and nuance to managing symptoms.

In the confluence of these efforts, lifestyle modifications, professional guidance, and supportive therapies, a strategy emerges—a multifaceted approach that acknowledges the complexity of managing anxiety and depression during menopause. It is a strategy that does not seek a singular solution but embraces a spectrum of interventions, each contributing to the delicate balance of mental and emotional health. This approach, woven with care and intention, offers symptom management and a pathway to a richer understanding of oneself, an opportunity to navigate menopause with a sense of agency and hope.

As we close this exploration of managing anxiety and depression within the broader narrative of menopause, we are reminded of the intricate interplay between body, mind, and spirit. The strategies outlined here, which encompass recognizing symptoms and seeking professional help, form part of a more extensive dialogue that encompasses not just the challenges of menopause but also the opportunities for growth and transformation it presents. With its focus on navigating the emotional and psychological complexities of menopause, this chapter sets the stage for continued exploration of well- being, leading us into discussions that further unravel the mysteries and magnificence of this pivotal life stage.

10 | Weaving Networks of Support

In the tapestry of managing menopause, the warp and weft of support systems play a pivotal role, a nuanced interplay between the individual and the collective. Within this intricate pattern, social media emerges as a vibrant thread, offering a platform where voices converge in a chorus of shared experiences, wisdom, and encouragement. Here, amidst the vast digital expanse, online communities become sanctuaries, spaces where the boundaries of time and geography blur, connecting individuals across the globe through the common thread of menopause. This digital congregation offers a unique blend of anonymity and accessibility. This juxtaposition fosters openness and honesty, allowing for the exchange of deeply personal narratives and insights without the weight of judgment.

10.1   Leveraging Social Media for Support

Finding Online Communities

Navigating the digital landscape to find these havens requires a blend of curiosity and discernment. Platforms vary, from the immediacy of Twitter, where hashtags like #MenopauseSupport or #WomenOver40 serve as beacons, guiding users to conversations and communities, to the structured forums of Facebook groups, where members gather under banners of shared interests or experiences. With its visual emphasis, Instagram offers a tapestry of personal stories and professional advice, captured in images and videos that speak to the multifaceted nature of menopause. Each platform holds potential, a gateway to communities where questions find answers, stories find listeners, and individuals find a sense of belonging.

The search for these communities might start with a simple query, a digital inquiry cast into the vastness of the internet. It evolves into a journey of connection, where each click and scroll brings individuals closer to finding their tribe. The key lies in using specific, targeted search terms—words that encapsulate the essence of one's quest for understanding and support. It's akin to setting a net with precision, ensuring that when it's drawn back, it's filled with meaningful connections rather than the residue of irrelevant content.

The Benefits of Online Support

The virtual embrace of these communities offers many benefits, such as a constellation of points of light on the sometimes dark night of menopause. Accessibility stands out; the internet is a portal that never closes, and its resources are available regardless of the hour. This round-the-clock access is particularly poignant during sleepless nights when menopause's hot flashes or insomnia hold sway. Anonymity, too, plays a crucial role, a cloak that grants the freedom to express vulnerabilities without fear of stigma or embarrassment. Within these digital spaces, stories and experiences flow freely, each post or comment a thread that weaves individuals into a larger, supportive tapestry.

Diversity enriches these online communities, introducing individuals to a broad spectrum of experiences and perspectives that might otherwise remain undiscovered. This exposure broadens understanding, challenges preconceptions, and fosters empathy, creating a richer, more inclusive conversation around menopause. The advice also finds fertile ground here, with recommendations from holistic remedies to medical interventions shared openly, each suggesting a potential avenue for relief and understanding.

Participating Respectfully

However, engagement in these communities carries a responsibility—a commitment to maintaining the sanctity of these spaces through respectful participation. Understanding and adhering to community guidelines is paramount, as well as a pact among members to uphold the values and norms that define the group's ethos. Privacy, too, demands vigilance, with personal boundaries respected and personal information guarded with care. This respectful engagement ensures that online communities remain havens of support, spaces where trust flourishes, and members feel safe to share and explore.

Avoiding Misinformation

In the vast ocean of information on the internet, misinformation lurks like an undertow, pulling the unwary into depths of confusion and uncertainty. Critical evaluation becomes a life-line, a skill that allows individuals to distinguish between credible advice and misleading claims. Verifying sources, cross-referencing information with reputable health sites, and consulting healthcare professionals before adopting new treatments or remedies are strategies that navigate around the pitfalls of misinformation, ensuring that the support and advice garnered from online communities enrich rather than mislead.

Visual Element: The Community Compass

A visual aid, "The Community Compass," offers a navigational tool for finding and engaging with online menopause support communities. This infographic outlines the steps for locating communities on various social media platforms, highlights the benefits of participation, and provides guidelines for respectful engagement and critical evaluation of information. A checklist accompanying the compass encourages reflection on one's goals and needs in seeking online support, ensuring that the journey into digital communities is purposeful and rewarding.

In the quest for support and understanding within the landscape of menopause, social media stands as a beacon, a digital gathering place where voices converge, stories intertwine, and individuals find solace and strength in the shared experience. Through careful navigation, respectful engagement, and vigilant evaluation, these online communities offer a rich tapestry of support, weaving together the individual and the collective in a vibrant network of connection and understanding.

10.2   Establishing Local Support Groups

In personal growth and adaptation, creating a local support group is a testament to the power of collective wisdom and shared resilience. Initiating such a group demands a vision and a committed heart, ready to weave together the diverse threads of individual experiences into a cohesive fabric of mutual support. While filled with potential, this endeavor unfolds through deliberate steps, each carefully considered to foster a space of inclusivity, understanding, and empowerment.

A local menopause support group begins with the spark of connection, an initial gathering of individuals drawn together by shared circumstances. Finding these initial members taps into the wellspring of personal networks, community bulletins, and local health clinics, each serving as a conduit for reaching out to those navigating the menopausal transition. Social media, too, plays a pivotal role, not as the destination but as a means to extend the invitation, casting a wide net to capture the interest of potential members. The essence of this initial phase is outreach, a gentle call to those who seek not just answers but camaraderie in the quiet moments of reflection.

With the foundation of membership beginning to solidify, attention turns to the structure of interaction, the rhythm, and the flow of meetings that will define the group's cadence.

The choice of meeting format—whether structured discussions, informal coffee meetups, or themed workshops— reflects not just the preferences of the group but the under- lying goals that bind its members. Some groups may find strength in the structured sharing of experiences, a round- table where each voice finds its moment in the sun. Others may lean towards the fluidity of informal gatherings, where conversation meanders like a river, touching on topics as varied as the individuals present. The decision on format involves a dialogue, a collective shaping of the group's path forward.

Setting an agenda for each meeting injects a measure of intentionality into the proceedings. This roadmap guides but does not bind. Topics might range from navigating healthcare options and understanding hormonal therapies to exploring holistic remedies and sharing lifestyle tips. The agenda acts as a scaffold, providing structure but allowing for the organic growth of discussion, ensuring that the group's time together is both meaningful and responsive to its members' evolving needs.

Collaboration with healthcare professionals introduces a layer of depth to the group's exploration, bridging the gap between personal experience and medical insight. Inviting guest speakers—be they gynecologists, therapists, or nutritionists—enriches the conversation, providing credibility and a broadened perspective. These sessions, whether framed as informal Q&A or structured presentations, offer a rare opportunity for direct engagement with experts, a chance to demystify aspects of menopause that often seem cloaked in complexity. The key lies in selecting professionals with expertise, genuine empathy, and understanding of menopause as a lived experience, ensuring that their contributions resonate with and empower group members.

However, a support group's vitality hinges not on something other than its inception or the caliber of its meetings but on its ability to sustain momentum over time. This sustainability is cultivated through a dynamic interplay of leadership, engagement, and activity. Rotating leadership roles democratizes the group, ensuring that every member feels a sense of ownership and investment in its direction. This rotation brings fresh perspectives, preventing stagnation and fostering a vibrant, evolving community.

Engaging members outside of meetings through social activities or shared projects strengthens the bonds formed within the group, weaving tighter the fabric of support. These activities, whether group walks, book clubs focused on women's health, or volunteering projects, extend the group's impact beyond the confines of its meetings, embedding it within the larger tapestry of community life.

Strategies for maintaining engagement and enthusiasm range from celebrating milestones—personal or group achievements—to incorporating feedback mechanisms that allow the group to adapt and respond to its members' shifting needs. Regular check-ins, whether through surveys or open discussions, ensure that the group remains relevant and responsive, a living entity that grows in alignment with the individuals it serves.

In this endeavor, creating and nurturing a local menopause support group lies a profound opportunity for transformation.

It is an undertaking that requires not just logistical planning but emotional investment and an openness to both giving and receiving support. Through the collective exploration of menopause, individuals find solace in understanding and a shared strength. This communal resilience transcends the challenges of this transition. In the shared stories, laughter, tears, and mutual encouragement, the group becomes more than the sum of its parts—a beacon of hope and empowerment for all who gather within its embrace.

10.3   The Role of Professional Support

In the intricate dance of managing menopause, the embrace of professional support acts not merely as a step but as a pivotal way, enriching the rhythm established by personal efforts and the solidarity found within community networks.

This layer of guidance, dispensed by therapists, counselors, or menopause specialists, introduces a depth of understanding and an arsenal of strategies tailored to the nuances of one's physiological and psychological experiences. The synergy between professional insight and the foundational support from personal and community networks crafts a holistic approach to menopause management, weaving a safety net that catches the complexities often overlooked by singular coping methods.

Seeking the right professional ally necessitates a diligent vetting process, akin to sifting through grains to find pearls of wisdom that resonate with personal needs and circumstances. This quest involves consultations, often starting within the circles of primary care providers or gynecologists who can offer referrals based on a deep understanding of one's medical history and current challenges. The venture might extend into interviews with potential therapists or specialists, sessions where questions flow freely, aiming to gauge the professional's familiarity with menopause-related issues, their approach to treatment, and their philosophy on integrating care across different spectrums of health. This dialogue ensures that the chosen professional possesses the requisite expertise and aligns with one's values and expectations, promising a partnership that enriches the journey through menopause.

Integrating professional advice with self-guided strategies and the wisdom gleaned from support groups fosters an environment where learning and adaptation flourish. Professionals bring to the table a wealth of knowledge about therapeutic interventions, from cognitive-behavioral techniques aimed at mitigating anxiety to physiological treatments that address the myriad of physical symptoms. This expert guidance complements the lifestyle adjustments, emotional coping strategies, and communal wisdom shared within support networks, creating a multi-layered approach to menopause management. This integration ensures a response to menopause that is as dynamic and multifaceted as the experience. A confluence of knowledge empowers individuals to navigate this transition with informed confidence.

Advocating comprehensive care emerges as a crucial theme. This narrative thread demands recognition of menopause as a holistic experience that intersects physical, emotional, and psychological health. This advocacy involves vocalizing needs and concerns and seeking professionals who view menopause through a lens that captures its complexity.

It's about pushing for a care model that doesn't fragment the individual into symptoms to be treated in isolation but sees them as a whole person navigating a significant life transition. This comprehensive approach underscores the importance of a support system that addresses the entirety of menopause's impact, ensuring that care strategies are as interconnected as the symptoms and experiences they aim to address.

In this layered approach to managing menopause, professional support is a pillar, complementing and enhancing personal and communal efforts. It offers a bridge between the individual's rich, experiential knowledge and the broader, evidence-based treatments and strategies that stem from years of research and practice. This fusion of personal insight, communal wisdom, and professional expertise crafts a resilient, informed, and adaptive response to menopause, embracing the transition as a series of challenges to overcome and an opportunity for growth, discovery, and empowerment.

As we close this exploration of professional support in the broader context of menopause management, we are reminded of the power of a multifaceted approach. It is a reminder that while menopause might be a universal experience, the journey is deeply personal, shaped by the unique interplay of one's body, mind, and circumstances. In concert with personal strategies and community wisdom, professional support offers a comprehensive response to this life transition, ensuring that each individual can navigate menopause with a sense of agency and well-being. This holistic approach not only addresses the immediate challenges of menopause but also lays the groundwork for a future where health and happiness continue to flourish.

A Strong Support System Is Exactly What You Need to Become Support for the Next Woman

Although it will take some effort on your behalf, small changes can lead to immense changes in your quality of life. And let's face it—you are worthy of a fulfilling life! Let's ensure we let other women know they are worthy too! Your opinions are an invaluable part of the next woman's support system!

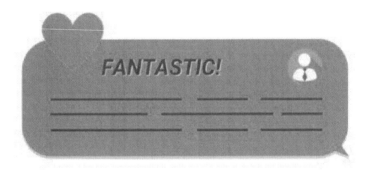

Honestly, I'm not only grateful for a couple of clicks you made to leave your review on Amazon, but I'm also really proud that you have become part of the movement to shake the stigma off menopause! Thank you so much and I can't wait to read how you are getting on!

Scan the QR code below

Conclusion

Hey there, excellent reader! We've been through quite the journey together, haven't we? From those first whispers of menopause to embracing a life filled with empowerment and laughter beyond it, I hope you've picked up from our little chats that menopause isn't just a phase to endure—it's an invitation to a grand adventure, a chance to rediscover your- self and, perhaps, to have a little fun along the way.

Remember, the key takeaways from our journey aren't just about understanding the nitty-gritty of hot flashes or why you suddenly feel like a polar bear in the Sahara. No, it's about recognizing the incredible transformation you're undergoing and harnessing it. It's about a holistic approach—melding mind, body, and spirit to dance through menopause with grace, a few good laughs, and maybe some chocolate (because why not?).

I can't stress enough the importance of keeping that beautiful mind of yours hungry for knowledge and advocacy.

Menopause research is ever-evolving, and with it, our understanding deepens. So, stay curious, my friend, and use your voice to elevate the conversation around menopause. Let's make it as familiar and comfortable a topic as discussing the weather (but infinitely more interesting).

Now, I'm passing the baton to you. Take these strategies, tips, and tales of triumph (and the occasional misstep) and weave them into the fabric of your own journey. Share the wisdom you've gathered far and wide. Remember, your menopause experience is as unique as you are—there's no one-size-fits-all here. Tailor what you've learned to suit your fabulous self, and don't be shy about seeking out or forging new support communities. After all, we're all in this together.

Your story doesn't end here. In fact, I'd like to get started. I'd love nothing more than for you to share your tales from the menopause frontier. Let's keep the conversation going—whether on social media, in cozy living room gatherings, or as part of a book club discussion. Your story is powerful; it's needed and could be the lighthouse for someone else navigating these waters.

Thank you, from the bottom of my heart, for joining me on this wild ride. Your willingness to dive into these pages, to explore, question, and maybe even chuckle at the quirks of menopause, means the world to me. Together, we're reshaping the narrative around this pivotal stage of life, making it one of empowerment, understanding, and, yes, even a bit of joy.

As we part ways (just from this book, mind you), I leave you with this: envision a future where menopause is not whispered about in hushed tones but celebrated as a rite of passage. A world where information flows freely, support networks are vast, and the journey through menopause is embraced with open arms and hearts. My dear reader, you are at the forefront of creating this beautiful future. So, step boldly, share generously, and live vibrantly. The best is yet to come.

With all my gratitude and warmest wishes for your journey ahead,

Annabel Wave

P.S. Remember, menopause might try to be the boss, but you, my dear, can write your own script. Let's make it a blockbuster.

References

⮀ National Library of Medicine. 2019. "Home - Books - NCBI." Nih.gov. 2019. https://www.ncbi.nlm.nih.gov/books/.

⮀ Estrogen vs. Progesterone: Functions in the Human Body https://www.healthline.com/health/womens-health/estrogen-vs-progesterone#:

⮀ Menopause - Things you can do - NHS https://www.nhs.uk/conditions/menopause/things-you-can-do/

⮀ Perimenopause - Symptoms and causes https://www.mayoclinic.org/diseases-conditions/perimenopause/symptoms-causes/syc-20354666

⮀ Nutrition in Menopausal Women: A Narrative Review - PMChttps://www.ncbi.nlm.nih.gov/pmc/articles/PMC8308420/ Exercise beyond menopause: Dos and Don'ts - PMC - NCBIhttps://www.ncbi.nlm.nih.gov/pmc/articles/PMC3296386/

⮀ Sleep Problems and Menopause: What Can I Do? https://www.nia.nih.gov/health/menopause/sleep-problems-and-menopause-what-can-i-do

⮀ 10 Natural Ways to Balance Your Hormones - Healthline https://www.healthline.com/nutrition/balance-hormones

⮀ Impact of Estradiol Variability and Progesterone on Mood

⮀ ...https://www.ncbi.nlm.nih.gov/pmc/articles/PMC7075107/ Mindfulness may ease menopausal symptoms https://newsnetwork.mayoclinic.org/discussion/mindfulness-may-ease-menopausal-symptoms/

⊃ North American Menopause Society (NAMS) - Focused on Providing Physicians, Practitioners & Women Menopause Information, Help & Treatment Insights. https://www. menopause.org/

⊃ How To Talk To Your Family About The Menopause https://www. mymenopausecentre.com/blog/how-to-talk-about-the-menopause/ My personal experience of the menopause - PMC https://www. ncbi.nlm.nih.gov/pmc/articles/PMC5325642/

⊃ Understanding the Implications of Society and Culture https:// www.pghr.org/post/menopause-understanding-the-implications- of-society-and-culture

⊃ Supporting someone through the menopause - NHS inform https://www.nhsinform.scot/healthy-living/womens-health/later- years-around-50-years-and-over/menopause-and-post-menopause-health/supporting-someone-through-the-menopause/

⊃ Building a Digital Community Around Menopause https:// redhotmamas.org/building-a-digital-community-around- menopause/

⊃ Menopause - Latest research and news https://www.nature.com/ subjects/menopause

⊃ Finding Reliable Health Information Online https://newsinhealth. nih.gov/2020/08/finding-reliable-health-information-online

⊃ North American Menopause Society (NAMS) - Focused on ... https://www.menopause.org

⊃ Clinical practice guidelines on menopause: An executive ... https:// www.ncbi.nlm.nih.gov/pmc/articles/PMC3785158/

⊃ 11 Natural Ways to Reduce Symptoms of Menopause https://www. healthline.com/nutrition/11-natural-menopause-tips

⊃ Benefits and risks of hormone replacement therapy (HRT) - NHS https://www.nhs.uk/medicines/hormone-replacement-therapy-hrt/benefits-and-risks-of-hormone-replacement-therapy-hrt/ Tracking Your Symptoms to Manage Menopause - Stella https:// www.onstella.com/the-latest/long-term-health/tracking-your-menopause-symptoms/

⊃ Menopause Is Finally Going Mainstream in Medicine https://time. com/6565057/menopause-treatment-symptoms-mainstream/ Omega-3 fatty acids for major depressive disorder ... https://www. ncbi.nlm.nih.gov/pmc/articles/PMC3195360/

⊃ Effects of Dietary Phytoestrogens on Hormones throughout

- ...https://www.ncbi.nlm.nih.gov/pmc/articles/PMC7468963/ How blood sugar can impact menopause symptoms https://www.levelshealth.com/blog/how-blood-sugar-can-impact-menopause-symptoms

- Hormonal Changes During Menopause and the Impact on

- ...https://www.ncbi.nlm.nih.gov/pmc/articles/PMC3984489/ Exercise beyond menopause: Dos and Don'ts - PMC - NCBIhttps://www.ncbi.nlm.nih.gov/pmc/articles/PMC3296386/

- Can I Balance Hormones With Pilates? - Healthnews https://healthnews.com/fitness/pilates/can-i-balance-hormones-with- pilates/#:

- Exercising in your 50s and beyond: Tips from a doctor and ... https://www.cnet.com/health/fitness/how-to-start-exercising-in- your-50s-and-beyond/

- High Physical Activity Level May Reduce Menopausal ... https://www.mdpi.com/1648-9144/55/8/466

- The effects of mindfulness-based interventions on anxiety

- ...https://www.ncbi.nlm.nih.gov/pmc/articles/PMC9869042/#:~ CBT can help with a range of menopausal symptoms, says NICEhttps://www.bmj.com/content/383/bmj.p2711#:

- The Effects of Perceived Stress and Attitudes Toward ... https://www.ncbi.nlm.nih.gov/pmc/articles/PMC3661682/ Psychosocial factors promoting resilience during the ... https://www.ncbi.nlm.nih.gov/pmc/articles/PMC7979610/

- Creating a Menopause Support Group https://executivesupportmagazine.com/menopause-support/

- Building a Digital Community Around Menopause https://redhotmamas.org/building-a-digital-community-around- menopause/

- The 2023 Practitioner's Toolkit for Managing Menopausehttps://www.tandfonline.com/doi/full/10.1080/13697137.2023.2258783 Holistic care of menopause: Understanding the framework https://www.ncbi.nlm.nih.gov/pmc/articles/PMC3555027/

- "Joycelyn Elders Quote." n.d. https://quotefancy.com/quote/1601267/Joycelyn-Elders-If-men-went-through-menopause-we-d-know-everything-about-it-but-we-still

Made in United States
Orlando, FL
16 September 2024

51606145R00112